THE BEST
IN TENT
CAMPING

VIRGINIA

SECOND EDITION

THE BEST IN TENT CAMPING

A GUIDE FOR CAR CAMPERS WHO HATE RVs, CONCRETE SLABS, AND LOUD PORTABLE STEREOS

VIRGINIA

SECOND EDITION

RANDY PORTER
with MARIE JAVINS

MENASHA RIDGE PRESS
BIRMINGHAM, ALABAMA

TABLE OF CONTENTS

VIRGINIA CAMPGROUNDS KEY

(Map on pages viii–ix)

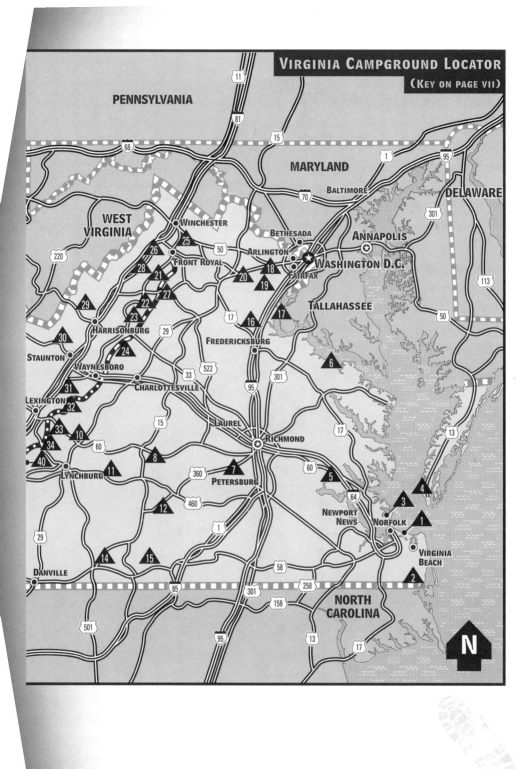

VIRGINIA CAMPGROUND LOCATOR
(KEY ON PAGE VII)

PENNSYLVANIA

MARYLAND

BALTIMORE

DELAWARE

WEST VIRGINIA

WINCHESTER

BETHESADA

ANNAPOLIS

ARLINGTON

WASHINGTON D.C.

FRONT ROYAL

FAIRFAX

TALLAHASSEE

HARRISONBURG

FREDERICKSBURG

STAUNTON

WAYNESBORO

CHARLOTTESVILLE

LEXINGTON

LAUREL

RICHMOND

LYNCHBURG

PETERSBURG

NEWPORT NEWS

NORFOLK

VIRGINIA BEACH

DANVILLE

NORTH CAROLINA

N

ACKNOWLEDGMENTS

THANKS TO all those who work to keep Virginia's parks and wild areas crown jewels of the Commonwealth.

—Randy Porter

THANKS TO my sister Lynn Javins of the Shenandoah Valley for co-piloting Henry the Ford Taurus through Virginia's western region. Thanks also to my father George Javins of Bath County for knowing exactly where to find the elusive Bubbling Springs—right down the road from Pig Run. Thanks to Michael Tunaley for his patience in brewing my morning coffee on the camp stove, regardless of the weather. He never did find an empty site on Skyline Drive in June. Kudos also to Linda and Frank Walcroft, my mother and her husband, who were kind enough to give me the keys to their Bryce cabin, where I wrote the updates to this book.

—Marie Javins

PREFACE

VIRGINIA IS A STATE, ACTUALLY A COMMONWEALTH, whose history and natural beauty are best described in superlatives. Her scenery varies from the coastal plain along the Atlantic Ocean and Chesapeake Bay to mountain ranges in the west and southwest. Her history parallels that of the New World, with the first settlers arriving in 1607, more U.S. presidents coming from Virginia than any other state, and the majority of Civil War battles being fought here. While the country was mired in the Great Depression in the 1930s, Virginia's public lands were the fortunate recipients of much of the labor of the Civilian Conservation Corps. As you travel about through the Old Dominion's federal- and state-managed public lands, you'll swim in lakes, hike on trails, and pitch your tent in areas that were born of one of the country's darkest periods.

I've lived in Virginia and explored its wooded countryside for three decades, and I still find myself overwhelmed by her glorious landscape and central role in the birth and growth of the United States. There's no better way to get to know the Old Dominion than by pitching a tent and camping out up close and personal. Walk her trails, fish in her streams, and sleep under her stars; and I'm convinced that you, too, will be taken by her charms.

—*Randy Porter*

THE BEST IN TENT CAMPING

VIRGINIA

SECOND EDITION

beautiful and achingly quiet, look for five stars in both of those categories. If you're more interested in a campground that has excellent security and cavernous campsites, look for five stars in the Spaciousness and Security categories. Keep in mind that these ratings are based somewhat on the subjective views of the authors and their sources.

BEAUTY

If this category needs explanation at all, it is simply to say that the true beauty of a campground is not always what you can see, but what you can't see. Or hear. Like a freeway. Or roaring motorboats. Or the crack, pop, pop, boom of a rifle range. An equally important factor for me on the beauty scale is the condition of the campground itself and to what extent it has been left in its natural state. Beauty also, of course, takes into consideration any fabulous views of mountains, water, or other natural phenomena.

SITE PRIVACY

No one who enjoys the simplicity of tent camping wants to be walled in on all sides by RVs the size of tractor trailers. This category goes hand in hand with the previous one because part of the beauty of a campsite has to do with the privacy of its surroundings. If you've ever crawled out of your tent to embrace a stunning summer morning in your skivvies and found several pairs of very curious eyes staring at you from the neighbor's picture window, you'll know what I mean. I look for campsites that are graciously spaced with lots of heavy foliage in between. You usually have to drive or even hike a little deeper into the campground complex for these.

SPACIOUSNESS

This is the category you toss the coin on—and keep your fingers crossed. I'm not as much of a stickler for this category because I'm happy if there's room to park the car off the main campground road, enough space to pitch a two- or four-man tent in a reasonably flat and dry spot, a picnic table for meal preparation, and a fire pit safely away from the tenting area. At most campgrounds, site spaciousness is sacrificed for site privacy and vice versa. Sometimes you get extremely lucky and have both. Don't be greedy.

QUIET

Again, this category goes along with the beauty of a place. When I go camping, I want to hear the sounds of nature. You know: birds chirping, the wind sighing, a surf crashing, a brook babbling. That kind of stuff. It's not always possible to control the noise volume of your fellow campers, so the closer you can get to natural sounds that can drown them out, the better. Actually, when you have a chance to listen to the quiet of nature, you'll find that it is really rather noisy. But what a lovely cacophony!

SECURITY

Quite a few of the campgrounds in this book are in remote and primitive places without on-site security patrol. In essence, you're on your own. Common sense is a great asset in these cases. Don't leave expensive outdoor gear or valuable camera equipment lying

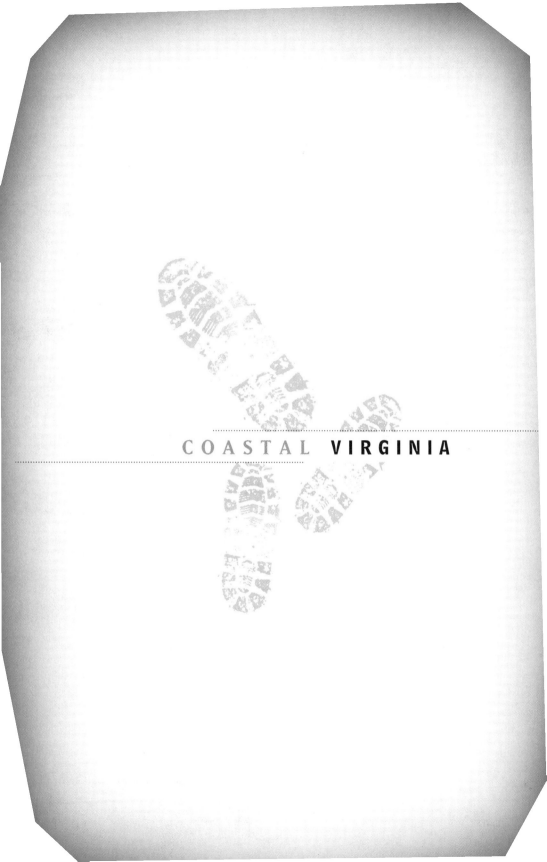

COASTAL VIRGINIA

KEY INFORMATION

ADDRESS: First Landing State Park
2500 Shore Drive
Virginia Beach, VA 23451

OPERATED BY: Virginia Department of Conservation and Recreation

INFORMATION: (757) 412-2300

WEB SITE: www.dcr.state.va.us/parks

OPEN: March 1–early December

SITES: 222

EACH SITE HAS: Picnic table, fire ring, and lantern pole

ASSIGNMENT: First come, first served

REGISTRATION: By phone, (800) 933-PARK; or on arrival. Reservations highly recommended.

FACILITIES: Water, hot showers, laundry, camp store, and pay phone

PARKING: One vehicle per site in addition to camping unit

FEE: $22 per night

ELEVATION: Sea level

RESTRICTIONS: Pets: On leash or in enclosed area; in swimming areas on leash with overnight guests only
Fires: In fire rings, stoves, or grills only
Alcohol: Prohibited
Vehicles: Up to 34 feet
Other: Do not damage any trees; bicycles only on park roads and the Cape Henry Trail; no motorized vehicles on trails; 14 of 30 days maximum stay; quiet hours 10 p.m.–8 a.m.

First Landing's trails can be accessed from the visitor center on the opposite side of US 60 from the campground. The 6-mile (point-to-point) Cape Henry Trail is extremely popular among bicyclists and stays busy, especially on weekends during the summer. Those out for a nice walk should keep that in mind and stick to the other 19 miles of trails that restrict bicycles. They range from the 0.3-mile Fox Run Trail to the 5-mile Long Creek Trail. Besides the usual coastal landscape that you might expect to find here where the Atlantic Ocean meets the Chesapeake Bay, the park is the northernmost location on the East Coast where you can see both subtropical and temperate plants growing together. It was included in the National Register of Natural Landmarks in 1965. As you walk through sand dunes that reach as high as 75 feet, don't be surprised to see Spanish moss hanging from bald cypress, wild olive, live oak, and beech trees.

Described as the park's most popular trail, the 1.5-mile Bald Cypress Trail starts from the visitor center and loops along boardwalks through cypress swamps complete with resident pileated woodpeckers and turtles sunning themselves on logs. The Long Creek Trail starts at the main park, beginning on the park's main road, and winds through salt marshes past osprey nests, great blue herons, and egrets stalking their prey.

False Cape State Park, the least-visited state park in Virginia, is located just a few miles away in the community of Sandbridge. False Cape's ranking can be attributed to its limited access, which is restricted to bicycle, boat, and foot. Additionally, day users can ride the electric tram in the summer and the low-impact, beach-oriented "Terra Gator" in the winter. Campers must hike, bike, or boat the 6 miles to the primitive campsites, which reward them with a secluded night in this near-pristine barrier peninsula.

NORTHWEST RIVER PARK

> *This land was once cultivated farmland, but shadier activities also went on here.*

NORTHWEST RIVER PARK'S 763 acres lie on the coastal plain near the southern border of Virginia. Those coming for the day or to spend a few nights will find peace and quiet with Indian Creek, Northwest River, and Smith Creek surrounding the park on three sides, and a 29-acre lake meandering through the middle of it. Don't worry about arriving unprepared to enjoy the water because paddleboats, johnboats, and canoes are all available for rent. You may also enjoy fishing in the stocked freshwater lake for bass, bluegill, crappie, catfish, and trout. This land was once cultivated farmland, but shadier activities also went on here. More than 30 sites for making moonshine have been found on the property, including four in the area known as Moonshine Meadow. Alcoholic beverages are currently prohibited.

After entering the park from Indian Creek Road, you'll arrive at the six-sided camp store and office next to the lake and boat rental area. Across the gravel road is the miniature golf course. After registering, take the gravel road to the right to reach the campground. The campground consists of 70 sites set out on two loops among a grove of towering oaks. The area is flat and shaded with little vegetative barrier between sites. They are spacious, however, with substantial distances between sites. Of the 19 non-electric tent sites, the most popular and private ones are 52, 53, 55, 58, 59, 61, 63, 65, 67, 68, and 70, which lie on the campground's outer edge. A backdrop of bamboo and hardwoods shields these sites but can also stifle breezes. This can be an important consideration when camping in

RATINGS

Beauty: ✿ ✿ ✿
Site privacy: ✿ ✿ ✿
Spaciousness: ✿ ✿ ✿
Quiet: ✿ ✿ ✿
Security: ✿ ✿ ✿
Cleanliness: ✿ ✿ ✿ ✿

MAP

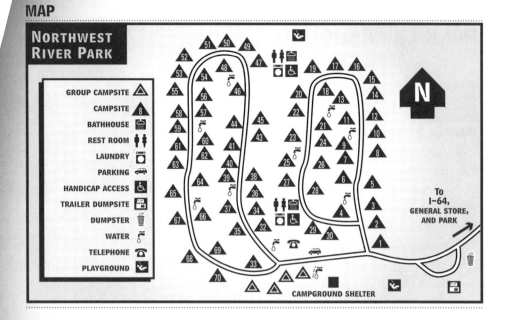

NORTHWEST RIVER PARK

GROUP CAMPSITE
CAMPSITE
BATHHOUSE
REST ROOM
LAUNDRY
PARKING
HANDICAP ACCESS
TRAILER DUMPSITE
DUMPSTER
WATER
TELEPHONE
PLAYGROUND

CAMPGROUND SHELTER

To
I-64,
GENERAL STORE,
AND PARK

GETTING THERE

From I-64, take the Battle-field Boulevard exit (VA 168) heading south. Continue 15 miles and turn left onto Indian Creek Road. Go 4 miles to the campground entrance.

trail loops around the fragrance garden for those who are either visually impaired or just enjoy a sweet-smelling garden. It's located next to the camp store. All of the park's trails are clearly marked and impeccably maintained.

In addition to self-guided activities, Northwest River Park offers instruction on its rope course for groups of eight to ten people. And turning your gaze skyward, you can learn about the heavens with the Backbay Amateur Astronomers, who meet in the evenings at the Equestrian Area.

ADDRESS: Newport News Park
13564 Jefferson
Avenue
Newport News, VA
23603

OPERATED BY: City of Newport
News Department
of Parks

INFORMATION: (757) 886-7912

WEB SITE: www.newport-news.
va.us/parks/

OPEN: Year-round

SITES: 188

EACH SITE HAS: Picnic table, fire
ring, and grill

ASSIGNMENT: Campers can choose
from available sites

REGISTRATION: By phone, (800) 203-
8322; or on arrival

FACILITIES: Laundry room, camp
store, hot showers,
water, flush toilets,
pay phones, and
drink machine

PARKING: 2 private vehicles
per campsite

FEE: $15.50 per night;
$17.50 with electric-
ity; $18 with electric-
ity and water

ELEVATION: 40 feet

RESTRICTIONS: Pets: On leash only
with proof of rabies
vaccination
Fires: Must be
attended; dead and
down wood may be
used for firewood
Other: Pitch tents
within 25 feet of the
pad with no more
than 2 tents per site
and only 1 camping
vehicle per site;
quiet hours 11 p.m.–
8 a.m.; length of stay
21 days within a 30-
day period from
April 1–October 31.

from other sites, and lie within a grove of mature hardwoods with some understory. Be sure to bring bug spray, as this is a low-lying area.

Camping at Newport News Park while sight-seeing the regional attractions is a popular and eco-nomical alternative to high-priced hotels. The park itself, however, offers several recreational options within walking and biking distance. These include the archery range, two 18-hole golf courses at Deer Run, an 18-hole disc golf course, and a 30-acre aeromodel flying field. Nature programs suitable for children and adults occur regularly in addition to the Children's Festival of Friends, the Newport News Fall Festival of Folklife, and the Celebration in Lights at Christmas when 450,000 lights transform the park into a magical place.

The park's bike path is popular among both cyclists and joggers. Its flat, sandy surface offers the opportunity for some leisurely exercise. Those look-ing to expand their adventure past the park's boundaries can take the turn for Washington's Headquarters located between the 2- and 3-mile markers. Taking this detour provides access to the Colonial National Historical Park at Yorktown where the last battle of the Revolutionary War was fought in 1781.

Hikers can stretch their legs on 30 additional miles of trails but bikers are restricted to the bike path and roads. Nature lovers should visit the trails located in the park's swampy area between the Deer Run Golf Course and the bike path just off the east-ern edge of the Lee Hall Reservoir.

Johnboats, canoes, and paddleboats are avail-able for rent should you want to fish for bass, pick-erel, pike, or perch or just want to take a leisurely ride around the 650 acres of freshwater provided by the park's two reservoirs.

Stop by the Interpretive Center to get a better idea of the park's place in the past and present. It

KIPTOPEKE STATE PARK

> *The drive across and under the bay coupled with the $10 one-way toll is a small price to pay for the tranquility that you'll find on the Eastern Shore.*

KIPTOPEKE STATE PARK is located at the southern end of Virginia's Eastern Shore just 3 miles from the Chesapeake Bay Bridge-Tunnel. Separated from the "mainland" of the Old Dominion by the 20-mile bridge-tunnel, the Eastern Shore is an entirely different world with a much slower pace than the one you left behind in Norfolk. The drive over and under the bay coupled with the $10 one-way toll is a small price to pay for the tranquility of the Eastern Shore. This 540-acre park offers 4,276 feet of beach frontage for swimming, surf casting, or just a leisurely stroll while watching the sunset.

After leaving US 13 and entering Kiptopeke (which translates to "big water"), you'll find the campground on the right just a short distance up the park's main road. The campsites are arranged in rows and vary from full hookups to no hookups and from open field to dense pine woods. The campsites get more wooded with higher numbers: 1–94 are mostly open and 95–141 are wooded (but offer minimal amenities). As you'd expect, the sea-level campground is flat, so there are options as to where to set up your tent within any given site. In choosing a temporary home site at Kiptopeke, however, keep in mind that woods can be both a plus and a minus when you're camping on the coast. It provides privacy from other campers, but the heavy growth of pines and underbrush also cut off welcome breezes that can cool a sultry summer day and push pesky, six-legged critters right past your site. If you neglected to pack your tent, you can rent a Kiptopeke yurt. Boardwalks from the campground

RATINGS

Beauty: ✿ ✿ ✿ ✿
Site privacy: ✿ ✿ ✿
Spaciousness: ✿ ✿ ✿
Quiet: ✿ ✿ ✿ ✿
Security: ✿ ✿ ✿
Cleanliness: ✿ ✿ ✿ ✿

MAP

KIPTOPEKE STATE PARK

SITES 111-121

SITES 121-141

SITES 95-110

INFORMATION

BATHHOUSE

REST ROOM

PARKING

TRAILER DUMPSITE

BEACH

BOAT RAMP

SITES 72-94

GROUP SITES

To SR 704

SITES 1-71

SHELTER

CHESAPEAKE BAY

GETTING THERE

From Norfolk, cross the Chesapeake Bay Bridge-Tunnel on US 13. After 3 miles turn left onto SR 704 until you reach the park entrance.

ADDRESS: Chippokes Plantation State Park
695 Chippokes Park
Road
Surry, VA 23883

OPERATED BY: Virginia Department
of Conservation
and Recreation

INFORMATION: (757) 294-3625

WEB SITE: www.dcr.state.va.us/
parks

OPEN: March–early
December

SITES: 32

EACH SITE HAS: Electricity, water,
picnic table, lantern
pole, fire ring, and
tent pad

ASSIGNMENT: Your choice

REGISTRATION: By phone, (800) 933-
PARK; or on arrival

FACILITIES: Flush toilets, hot
showers, drink
machines, and pay
phone

PARKING: 1 vehicle in addition
to camping unit at
campsite; overflow
parking at swim-
ming pool

FEE: $23 per night

ELEVATION: 100 feet

RESTRICTIONS: Pets: On leash and
not allowed in swim-
ming areas or rest
rooms; $3 surcharge
Fires: In fire rings,
stoves, or grills only
Alcohol: Prohibited
Vehicles: Up to 40
feet
Other: Do not carve,
chop, or damage any
live trees; keep
noise at a reasonable
level; no boat
launching at park;
length of stay no
more than 14 days in
a 30-day period.

important criterion in site selection for you, take a look at sites 8, 12, 14, 17, 19, 23–26, and 32.

The park has 3.5 miles of paved trails for hikers and bikers. Scheduled nature activities include guided fossil walks along the James River waterfront and canoe trips on the quiet streams that teem with both indigenous and migratory wildlife of the lower James River.

If you're looking to venture farther afield and continue your colonial history lessons, head over to Scotland Wharf (about 5 miles away). From there take the 15-minute ferry ride to Jamestown. Colonial Williamsburg is a scant 10 miles away on the Colonial Parkway, perhaps one of the most beautiful roads in America. Another 15 miles on the parkway will take you to the Yorktown Battlefield, where the Revolutionary War ended. From the north side of the James River, those less interested in history and more intent on contemporary entertainment can head for the roller coasters of Busch Gardens or the water slides of Water Country USA.

Chippokes and I go back to the early 1970s when, as an undergraduate at the College of William and Mary, I would venture across the James River and pedal around the quiet, rural back roads of Surry County. Surry seems to have changed very little in the intervening twenty-some years, so road cycling along the county's little-traveled roads is still an enjoyable activity while visiting Chippokes.

An especially fun time to visit is in July when the annual Pork, Pine, and Peanut Festival is taking place at Chippokes, where you can sample some of the best pork and peanut dishes; enjoy down-home bluegrass, country, and gospel music; and admire the craftsmanship of more than 230 artisans. The park's facilities are presently being expanded with the addition of several campsites, pool concessions, new water infrastructure, and the restoration of historic

WESTMORELAND STATE PARK

> *You'll undoubtedly want to explore Westmoreland between April and the end of November when its three campgrounds are open.*

WESTMORELAND STATE PARK, located on Virginia's rural Northern Neck peninsula, is best known for its views of the Potomac from the Horsehead Cliffs. Additionally, the park is positioned between the birthplaces of both George Washington and Robert E. Lee, its campgrounds providing history buffs with an economical alternative to hotels.

The campgrounds are closed in the off-season but the 1,299-acre park itself is open. Set aside the Horsehead Cliffs and instead stroll the sandy paths to view the seasonal holly and ilex opaca that stands out against the somber deciduous oak, hickory, and beech forest. Festooned with bright red berries set against shining green leaves, the holly branches sing of the season and fill the woods with cheer.

Established in 1936, Westmoreland was one of Virginia's first six state parks. Apart from the holiday season, it's best to explore Westmoreland between March and the end of November when its three campgrounds are open. After turning off VA 3 in the village of Baynesville onto VA 347, it's a mile to the park's contact station. Continuing, you'll arrive first at campground C, on the right, where the park road's two lanes divide around a wooded median strip. The first of these 40 sites alternates on either side of the campground road until a loop forms, housing sites 14–40. It's on this loop that campers desiring a little privacy will want to pitch their nylon getaway. Site 34 is particularly well secluded from the beaten path. It is also adjacent to the 2.5-mile Turkey Neck Trail, which loops around the eastern section of the park.

RATINGS

Beauty: ✪ ✪ ✪ ✪
Site privacy: ✪ ✪ ✪
Spaciousness: ✪ ✪ ✪
Quiet: ✪ ✪ ✪
Security: ✪ ✪ ✪
Cleanliness: ✪ ✪ ✪ ✪

MAP

WESTMORELAND STATE PARK

POTOMAC RIVER

CONVENIENCE STORE

INFORMATION

INFORMATION

N

BATHHOUSE	
REST ROOM	
PARKING	
TRAILER DUMPSITE	
BOAT RAMP	
SWIMMING	

SITES B28-51

SITES B1-27

37

CABINS 26-31

SITES A1-38

SITES C1-40

GETTING THERE

From I-95, take VA 3 at Fredericksburg and drive for 40 miles to the town of Baynesville. Turn left onto VA 347 to enter the park.

Cliffs outings. Kids of all ages will enjoy hunting for sharks' teeth dating from nearly 23 million years ago at the base of the cliffs.

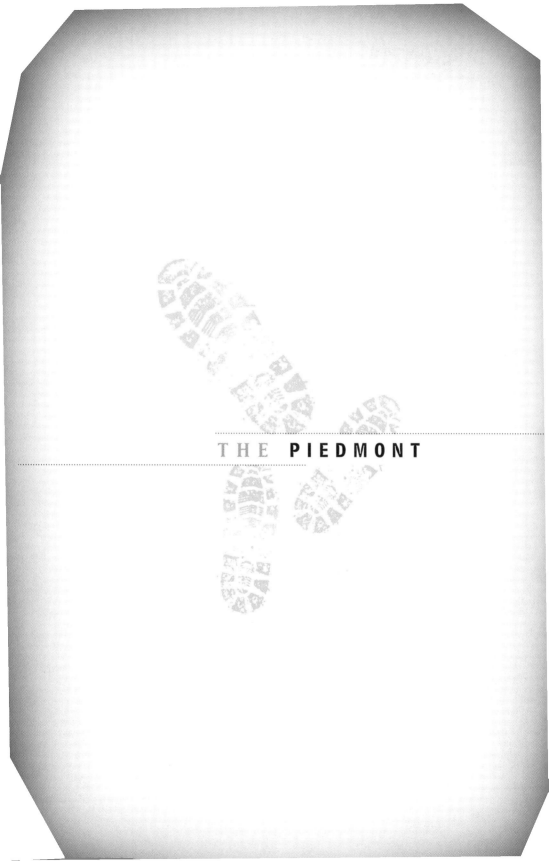

THE **PIEDMONT**

KEY INFORMATION

ADDRESS: Pocahontas State
Park
10301 State Park Road
Chesterfield, VA
23838-4713

OPERATED BY: Virginia Department
of Conservation
and Recreation

INFORMATION: (804) 796-4255

WEB SITE: www.dcr.state.va.us/
parks

OPEN: March–early
December

SITES: 65

EACH SITE HAS: Picnic table, lantern
pole, fire ring, and
electric and water
hookups

ASSIGNMENT: First come, first
served

REGISTRATION: (800) 933-PARK or on
arrival

FACILITIES: Flush toilets, hot
showers, pay
phones, and drink
machines

PARKING: 1 vehicle and 1
camping unit per
site; oveflow near
contact station

FEE: $23 per night

ELEVATION: 200 feet

RESTRICTIONS: Pets: $3 per night, on
leash only
Fires: Grills, camp
stoves, or designated
fire rings only
Alcohol: Prohibited
Vehicles: Up to 40
feet
Other: Do not dam-
age trees; no motor-
ized vehicles on
trails; swimming
only in designated
area; no gasoline
motors on lake; no
more than 14 days in
a 30-day period.

hillside along Swift Creek has given way to a larger facility with full electric and water hookups. While the quaintness of the former setting has been lost to us tent campers with the new, more RV-friendly campground, there are numerous sites that offer privacy and solitude. The preponderance of mature hardwoods helps maintain a feeling of sanctuary.

After turning off Beach Road at the park's entrance, you'll drive down the wide forest-lined park road for a mile before reaching the contact station, after which you'll see the campground entrance on the right. The 65 campsites are situated along the main access road and loops A, B, and C against a dense backdrop of mature oaks with shorter holly and pine trees.

Hikers and mountain bikers can enjoy more than 25 miles of forest roads and trails that meander throughout the park. Some trails circle the 24-acre Beaver Lake, while others wind through the hardwood forest. Those out for a leisurely stroll will enjoy the 2.5-mile Beaver Lake Trail, and the 3.2-mile Old Mill Bicycle Trail offers an easy pedal through the park. Fat-tire bicyclists looking for a greater challenge will head for the three newly constructed technical single-track trails that were built as a joint effort between Pocahontas State Park and Mountain Bike Virginia bike club. Be sure to pick up copies of the Pocahontas Park Guide and Bike Trails Guide. There are also 9 miles of bridal paths for equestrian use on a BYOH (Bring Your Own Horse) basis.

Pocahontas State Park is also home to the Civilian Conservation Corps Museum. From 1933 to 1942, FDR responded to the Great Depression by creating an "army with shovels" that planted two billion trees, built roads, bridges, trails, and 800 state parks. The CCC Museum is housed in an original CCC building. Exhibits include letters, artifacts, photographs and historic mementos that pay tribute

BEAR CREEK LAKE
STATE PARK

" *Visitors can choose from an array of outdoor activities, including sunbathing, swimming, and practicing on the state park system's only archery range.* "

BEAR **CREEK LAKE STATE PARK,** unique for its archery range, is a small park located near Richmond in Central Virginia's Cumberland State Forest. It features a variety of outdoor and water activities to keep both vacationers and urban refugees happy. The park's three campgrounds, designated A, B, and C, are nestled in the shade of mature towering sweet gum, oak, and tulip polar trees. There are 24 sites restricted to tents only.

Campground A sits on a hillside overlooking 40-acre Bear Creek Lake just behind the camp office. The campground host's site is adjacent to the picnic shelter at site A25. The sites are fairly close together. If given a choice, try to snag sites 10, 11, or 17, as they hug the lake. The small loop encompassing sites A5–A13 has no hookups and is suited to self-sufficient tent campers.

Campground B, with electric and water hookups, is the busiest of the three. It is located across the road from the camp office and features 20 sites on a single loop under a roof of hardwoods. The sites are close together and the loop lacks a bathhouse.

Tent camping is popular in Campground C as the sites lack hookups. The single campsite loop is flat and has its own bathhouse. Campground C contains ten sites with numbers 8 and 10 being the most private. The quarter-mile Running Cedar Trail is just across the road and provides access to the Lakeside Trail and swimming beach.

Bear Creek Lake State Park's archery range is the only one in the Virginia state park system. Ten bale targets bearing faces of assorted big game—such

RATINGS

Beauty: ✪ ✪ ✪ ✪
Site privacy: ✪ ✪
Spaciousness: ✪ ✪ ✪
Quiet: ✪ ✪
Security: ✪ ✪ ✪
Cleanliness: ✪ ✪ ✪ ✪

MAP

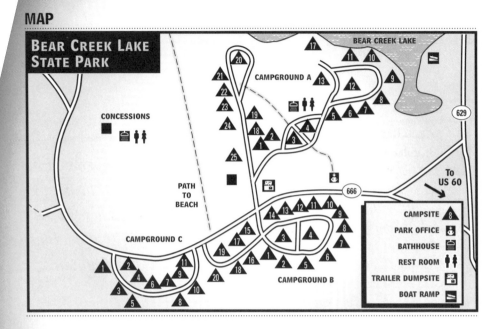

BEAR CREEK LAKE STATE PARK

CONCESSIONS

BEAR CREEK LAKE

CAMPGROUND A

PATH TO BEACH

CAMPGROUND C

CAMPGROUND B

To US 60

629

666

CAMPSITE	8
PARK OFFICE	
BATHHOUSE	
REST ROOM	
TRAILER DUMPSITE	
BOAT RAMP	

GETTING THERE

From US 60 east of Cumberland, go west on SR 622 and then south on SR 629 to the park entrance.

able). The relatively new Cumberland Multi-Use Loop Trail is fairly flat with the exception of a few sections. Parking is located next to the archery range. Although a linear rather than a loop trail, all points of the Willis River Trail are within 10 miles of Bear Creek Lake State Park and can be accessed from intersections with county and state forest roads. Also located near the park in Cumberland State Forest is a ten-station sporting clay range.

Between Memorial Day and Labor Day, Bear Creek Lake State Park also offers campfire talks and sing-alongs, night hikes, nature walks, children's programs, and slideshows.

ADDRESS: Fairy Stone State
Park
967 Fairystone Lake
Drive
Stuart, VA 24171

OPERATED BY: Virginia Department
of Conservation
and Recreation

INFORMATION: (276) 930-2424

WEB SITE: www.dcr.state.va.us/
parks

OPEN: March–early
December

SITES: 51

EACH SITE HAS: Picnic table, fire
grill, and water and
electric

ASSIGNMENT: First come, first
served

REGISTRATION: By phone, (800) 933-
PARK; or at camp-
ground on arrival

FACILITIES: Flush toilets, hot
showers, pay phone,
and drink machines
(by swimming
beach)

PARKING: 1 vehicle in addition
to camping unit;
additional parking a
half-mile away

FEE: $23 per night

ELEVATION: 1,240 feet

RESTRICTIONS: Pets: On leash and
attended; additional
fee charged per
night
Fires: Confined to
camp stoves and fire
rings
Alcohol: Public use
prohibited
Vehicles: Up to 30
feet
Other: No cutting or
marring of vegeta-
tion; length of stay
no more than 14
days in a 30-day
period.

cious use of a file will bring out one of several shapes in which they form. Should you come up empty-handed, however, Haynes Store offers a good selection at reasonable prices.

Fairy Stone was one of the six original parks in Virginia's park system in 1936. Its 4,868 acres made it the largest then, and it is still one of the largest today. After passing the 168-acre Fairy Stone Lake and beachfront on the left, you'll arrive at the contact station and the park office to the left of it. Straight ahead is the visitor center, where you'll want to stop to see the extensive collection of fairy stones as well as information about the local history and plant and animal life. Bear right at the visitor center and continue a short distance up the road to the entrance to the campground on the left.

The campground lies on one of many hilltops in the foothills of the Blue Ridge Mountains. The 51 sites, all with electric and water hookups, enjoy the shade of a pine grove dotted with scattered oaks. Most of the campsites have sand tent pads, with the exception of several pull-throughs. The single loop is located in the center of the park off local roads. A dense barrier of pines and hardwoods surrounds the campground. Thick stands of wild rhododendron grow throughout the park; an especially large one is across from the picnic area leading up to the campground.

Fairy Stone State Park features several hiking trails that range in length and degree of challenge from the 0.9-mile Beach Trail, which leads from site 28 to the lake and beach, to the orange-blazed Little Mountain Falls Trail. This 4.2-mile trail is accessible just across the road from the campground via the gated 2.1-mile Mountain View Hiking and Bicycle Trail. If you plan to hike, pick up one of the park's Stuart's Knob and Little Mountain Trail Systems Guides.

JAMES RIVER
STATE PARK

> *There is no privacy or undergrowth between riverfront sites, but while campers must view their neighbors, the views of the river can't be beat.*

JAMES RIVER STATE PARK opened in 1999 and is still in its infancy. It's one of the newest state parks in Virginia, having started with the purchase of land with funds from the 1992 General Obligation Bond. Its lack of camping amenities puts the two campgrounds in the "primitive" category, but for those who might not find the clean vault toilets appealing, rest assured that flushing toilets are available at the park's day-use area.

The park's canoe-in campsites are a major draw here, but James River also features three fishing ponds and picnic areas, along with 20 miles of trails for hikers, bikers, and equestrians.

Twenty-two sites sit near the James River at the canoe landing. RVs of up to 30 feet can be accommodated at some sites including nine riverfront drive-in sites, but there are several shaded tent-only sites along the river, just down a soft grassy bank. Campers must carry their gear around 40 feet from gravel parking spots to assigned tent sites. There is no privacy or undergrowth between sites, but while campers must view their neighbors, the views of the river can't be beat. Park planners hope to add RV sites with electrical and water hookups within a few years. There are five horse-camping sites and six stalls across the meadow from the Canoe Landing sites.

The riverside campground is the star camping attraction at James River State Park, with its landing where canoes can be launched from camper's front yards at Dixon Landing. Nearby Branch Pond Campground is located in an idyllic, secluded forest. Campers searching for scenic privacy or lake

RATINGS

Beauty: ✪ ✪ ✪ ✪
Site privacy: ✪ ✪
Spaciousness: ✪ ✪ ✪ ✪
Quiet: ✪ ✪ ✪
Security: ✪ ✪
Cleanliness: ✪ ✪ ✪

MAP

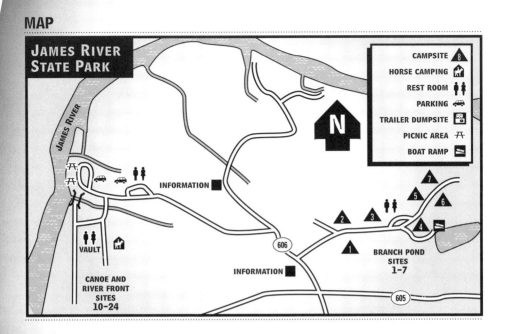

GETTING THERE

From US 60 near Amherst, head north on SR 605 at the James River Bridge. Travel 7 miles, then turn left onto SR 606.

the honor board. Walk-ins may not get a site, but Holliday Lake State Park has 30 sites nearby for those who find themselves site-less.

aquatic exploration. A Virginia fishing license is required to fish at Holliday Lake. The sandy beach-front swimming area offers a great way to cool off during the summer's heat or have lunch alfresco in the shady, lakefront picnic area.

Besides swimming, fishing, and boating, another attraction here is the trailhead for the 12-mile Carter Taylor Loop Trail, which starts inside the park across from the campground. After quickly leaving the park and entering the surrounding 19,535-acre Appomattox-Buckingham State Forest, the CT Loop Trail utilizes state forest and state roads as well as the occasional stretch of single-track. Pick up a copy of the Carter Taylor Loop Trail brochure, which shows the route of the multi-use trail open to hikers, bicyclists, and equestrians.

There are also shorter trails within the park's boundaries including the 0.75-mile Dogwood Ridge Trail and the 5-mile Lakeshore Nature Trail. The Appomattox-Buckingham State Forest is Virginia's largest with a considerable network of woods roads that are open to hikers, bikers, and equestrians. Those venturing out into the state forest should get a Forest Service map to stay oriented on the Carter Taylor as well as for assistance in developing additional routes through the rolling countryside. Holliday Lake also features the unique Sunfish Aquatic trail, a self-guided adventure that requires a boat to navigate.

Civil War buffs will not want to miss the opportunity to visit the Appomattox Court House National Historic Park where Confederate General Robert E. Lee surrendered to Union General Ulysses S. Grant to end the Civil War, also known here in Virginia as the War of Northern Aggression. Lee's Army of Northern Virginia, weary and tattered, passed approximately 1.5 miles from the present park site en route to the final battles of the war. The park encompasses some 1,800 acres of rolling

TWIN LAKES
STATE PARK

The 6,970-acre Prince Edward–Gallion State Forest surrounds the park and offers an array of gated forest roads that are open to hikers and bikers.

LOCATED NEAR **FARMVILLE** in a shady area of mature hardwoods, Twin Lakes State Park is named for Goodwin Lake and Prince Edward Lake. The two lakes were in separate racially segregated parks that began operations in 1939 and continued in this fashion until the Civil Rights Act passed in 1964. The two integrated parks then operated separately until merging into one 425-acre park in 1976. The name was changed to Twin Lakes State Park in 1986. The park's main road and the 0.25-mile Between the Lakes Trail connect the two units. Facilities at Goodwin Lake are available for individual camping, picnicking, and swimming. The eastern shore of Prince Edward Lake, meanwhile, features group camping, a lodge, and cabins at the Cedar Crest Conference Center. The conference center is available by reservation only, with cabin rentals possible when not previously booked by groups.

After entering the park off of SR 629, you'll find the campground located opposite the contact station. It consists of a large loop with a smaller loop at the rear. All of the sites are spacious, include water and electric hookups, and are set against a dense wooded background that provides ample shade during the summer. Sites 10 and 12, located at the back of the smaller loop that encompasses sites 6–15, are the most private of all. Tent pads are gravel, so pack a ground cloth for your tent and sleeping pad.

The day-use area at Goodwin Lake includes the 1.5-mile Goodwin Lake Nature Trail, sandy beach, picnic tables, and a playground. The concession area, aka "The Spot," is also located near here, and

RATINGS

Beauty: ✫ ✫ ✫
Site privacy: ✫ ✫
Spaciousness: ✫ ✫ ✫
Quiet: ✫ ✫ ✫
Security: ✫ ✫ ✫
Cleanliness: ✫ ✫ ✫

MAP

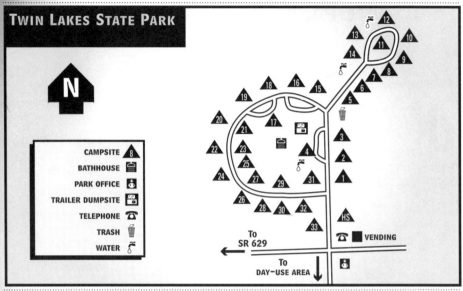

TWIN LAKES STATE PARK

CAMPSITE	
BATHHOUSE	
PARK OFFICE	
TRAILER DUMPSITE	
TELEPHONE	
TRASH	
WATER	

To SR 629

To DAY-USE AREA

VENDING

GETTING THERE

From Richmond, drive west for approximately 50 miles on US 360 through the town of Burkeville. Turn right onto SR 613 at the sign for Twin Lakes, and then turn right after a mile onto SR 629. Turn left into the campground entrance after driving 2 miles.

Petersburg to Appomattox, so you can tune to 1610 AM on your car radio to learn more about the events and battle that ended the Civil War.

The park is spread out over 1,248 densely wooded acres of Virginia pine, American beech, and juniper, which provide a back-to-nature feel while keeping the lake out of sight. The campground, visitor center, and boat launch and swimming area are situated on three separate peninsulas, so access from one to the other is best handled by car. You can also reach the water by way of the trails, which range in length from the 0.5-mile Lake View Trail to the 1.9-mile Chestnut Ridge. Just outside the gated entrance to the visitor center is a kiosk and trailhead for the 1.3-mile Turtle Island Trail. The 0.5-mile Beechwood Trail is accessible from the dump station located next to the campground entrance. All of these trails provide easy to moderate excursions for hikers of average physical condition.

After entering the park from SR 626, you'll see the park office on the right past the contact station. Turn left onto Interpretive Trail Road across from the office, and then turn left onto Overnight Road. You'll find the campground on the right with overflow parking across the road. The campground consists of dual loops on which 50 sites are located. Sites 16–26, 27–35, and 42–47 lack hookups and are set off a short distance in the woods. Access to these sites requires a short walk from your car, but the additional privacy is worth it.

The other sites are located along the campground loop and set fairly close together. All sites are close to the new bathhouse, which is positioned in the center of the lower loop. Its flushing toilets and hot showers replaced the vault toilets in 2003. Like the rest of the park, the campground is set among a mixture of conifers and deciduous trees offering plentiful shade. Twenty en-suite rental cabins are located nearby and feature docks and first-come, first-served slips. With Smith Mountain Lake's popularity as a destination for bass anglers,

STAUNTON RIVER
STATE PARK

> *While Occoneechee State Park may be the first choice for boaters and anglers, the seclusion that Staunton River offers is well worth the 45-minute drive from Occoneechee.*

STAUNTON RIVER STATE PARK is located on a peninsula upstream from Occoneechee State Park at the narrow end of Buggs Island Lake, also known as the John H. Kerr Reservoir. The park and adjacent river are named for pre–Revolutionary War commander Captain Henry Staunton, whose contingent of soldiers kept early settlers safe from Native American attacks. This section of the Dan River became known as Captain Dan's River and later the Staunton River. It became an important route for transporting tobacco from the large plantations that were built in this southernmost section of Virginia. Unfortunately, most were destroyed during the Civil War. This 1,597-acre park was one of the original six in Virginia's fledgling state park system. It opened in 1936, with many of the buildings constructed by the Civilian Conservation Corps from 1933–1935. Kerr Dam's opening in 1952 created the 48,000-acre Buggs Island Lake.

While nearby Occoneechee State Park may be the first choice for boaters and anglers, the seclusion that Staunton River offers is well worth the 45-minute drive from Occoneechee. VA 344 forms the main park road before terminating at the end of the peninsula. Shortly after passing the contact station, you'll see the sign for Staunton River's Campground on the left. Turn in here and enter the intimate figure eight over which the 49 sites are spread around a bathhouse in the center. Only 14 of these are standard sites without electric and water hookups, so when things get busy you're likely to have RVs for neighbors. The campground lies in a

RATINGS

Beauty: ✿ ✿ ✿
Site privacy: ✿ ✿
Spaciousness: ✿ ✿
Quiet: ✿ ✿ ✿
Security: ✿ ✿ ✿ ✿
Cleanliness: ✿ ✿ ✿ ✿

MAP

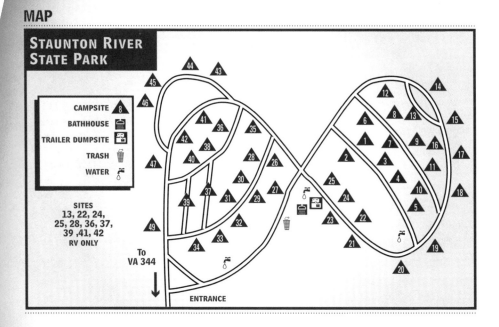

GETTING THERE

From US 58 along the southern border of Virginia, follow US 360 east for 18 miles from South Boston. Turn right and continue 10 miles on VA 344 to the park entrance.

road line has re-opened as a 0.8-mile walking trail from Staunton River bridge to Randolph.

ADDRESS: Occoneechee State
Park
1192 Occoneechee
Park Road
Clarksville, VA
23927

OPERATED BY: Virginia Department
of Conservation
and Recreation

INFORMATION: (434) 374-2210

WEB SITE: www.dcr.state.va.us/
parks

OPEN: March 1–early
December

SITES: 88

EACH SITE HAS: Picnic table, fire
grill, and lantern
pole

ASSIGNMENT: On arrival as
available

REGISTRATION: By phone, (800) 933-
PARK; or on arrival

FACILITIES: Flush toilets, hot
showers, and laun-
dry sinks

PARKING: At campsites, trail-
heads, and boat
landing

FEE: $18 per night; $23
with electric and
water

ELEVATION: 350 feet

RESTRICTIONS: Pets: Must be on a 6-
foot or shorter leash;
$3 per night
Fires: Confined to
camp stove or fire
ring
Alcohol: Public use
or display is prohib-
ited
Vehicles: Up to 30
feet
Other: Length of
stay no more than 14
days in a 30-day
period; limit 6 peo-
ple per campsite.

divided among his children and slaves. Eventually the mansion was sold outside the family and later burned to the ground in 1898.

After leaving US 58 to enter the park, you'll drive down VA 364, the park's main road. Turn left after the contact station and continue a short distance until you reach campground B on the right-hand side. There are 88 sites spread out over campgrounds B and C. The area once known as campground A was absorbed into the adjacent Occoneechee Wildlife Management Area. Campground B is divided with 52 sites designated for tent camping. The rest have hookups for RVs.

Park designers creatively arranged the tent-camping area to maximize privacy and excellent waterfront vistas. As you drive around the outer tent-camping loop looking for a good space, check out the sites numbered B31–B46 for the ideal combination. Many of the best sites are a short walk from their designated parking areas and set into the hillsides overlooking the lake or dense woods of oak, pine, and cedar. Tent camping sites at campground B are generally isolated from each other and offer better-than-average distance from the road.

The entrance to campground C is farther down the park road on the right after you pass the 0.8-mile Big Oak Nature Trail. Many of the 35 sites located along dual loops on a small peninsula offer electric and water hookups and are located close together. Campground C is more RV-oriented and would be the second choice for tent campers looking for quiet and privacy.

Besides the great fishing and boating that the John H. Kerr Reservoir has to offer, campers can enjoy a leisurely walk along the park's color-blazed trail system located between the contact station and entrance road to campground B. The trails range in length from the 1.2-mile Old Plantation Interpretive

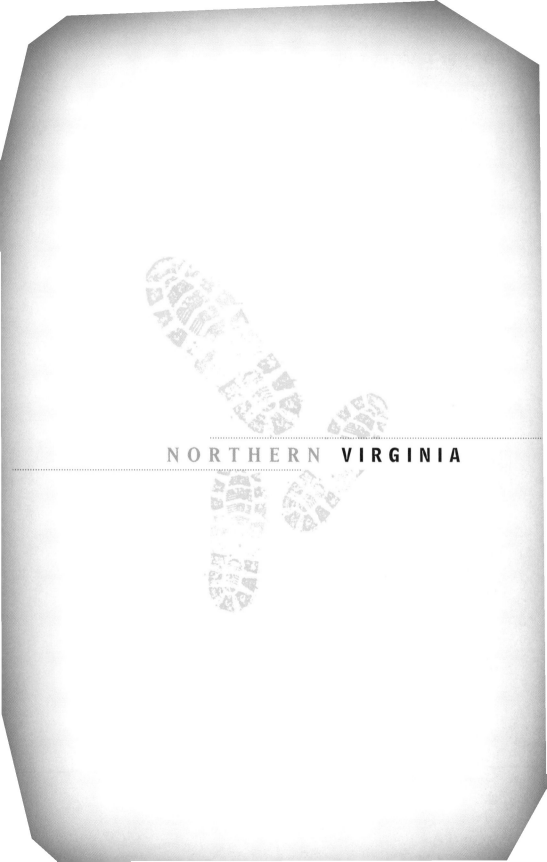

NORTHERN **VIRGINIA**

KEY INFORMATION

ADDRESS: Prince William Forest Park
P.O. Box 209
Triangle, VA 22172-0209

OPERATED BY: National Park Service

INFORMATION: (703) 221-7181

WEB SITE: www.nps.gov/prwi

OPEN: Year-round

SITES: 80

EACH SITE HAS: Picnic table, grill, and lantern pole

ASSIGNMENT: First come, first served

REGISTRATION: Self-registration on site

FACILITIES: Water, flush toilets, shower in B loop, and bike rack

PARKING: 2 vehicles per site, additional vehicles park at campground entrance

FEE: $5 entry; $15 camping

ELEVATION: 350 feet

RESTRICTIONS: Pets: Must be on leash shorter than 6 feet
Fires: Must be in grills; BYO firewood, no collecting deadwood
Alcohol: Allowed at campsite
Vehicles: Up to 32 feet
Other: Quiet hours 10 p.m.– 6 a.m.; site capacity, 2 tents and 6 people; 14-day stay limit; fireworks, firearms, and weapons are prohibited.

from the visitor center along the paved scenic drive. Plan to have $10 per night camping fee in exact change ready so that once you've pitched your tent, you're good to go. Once you've made it to this oasis, you'll not want to use your car again until it's time to go.

The Oak Ridge Campground consists of three loops, A, B, and C, with nary a hookup among the 80 sites. RVers will have motored to Travel Trailer Village on the other side of the park, so you're not likely to be running up against somebody's Minnie Winnie. Collecting firewood is prohibited in the interest of rebuilding topsoil and providing wildlife habitat. Campers must bring their own firewood from outside the park.

The overall terrain is rolling, but the campground itself is private, flat, and heavily wooded with second-growth oaks and some small pines. Sites vary in size from spacious in loops A and B to the extremely spacious walk-in sites in loop C. The campground rarely fills up. Some use this campground as a relatively inexpensive way to explore Washington, but my feeling is that it's too beautiful and natural a setting to park and drive away. There are several Northern Virginia campgrounds that are closer to D.C., but if you opt to use Prince William as your base camp for urban exploration, avoid rush hour on I-95 by taking the Virginia Rail Express from nearby Rippon or Quantico to D.C.'s Union Station.

Opportunities for bikers and hikers abound at this park, so once you've settled into your site, just leave your car until it's time to go home. Some 37 miles of well-blazed hiking trails with varied lengths and degrees of difficulty wind through the beech, holly, and oak forest. The best place to start might be the 1-mile Farms to Forest Trail (with a possible 2.7-mile extension through beaver habitat), which begins right at the campground entrance. From the

POHICK BAY
REGIONAL PARK

> *Even landlubbers will find these 150 campsites great places to sleep under the trees.*

POHICK WAS NAMED by Algonquin Indians to aptly describe this area as the "water place." With its marina, boat launch, and boat storage facilities, Pohick Bay Regional Park offers a year-round haven for boaters looking for access to the Potomac River, just 25 miles south of Washington, D.C., in Fairfax County. Those without a boat can choose from the park's rental fleet of pedal boats, sailboats, and johnboats. Even landlubbers will find Pohick Bay's 150 campsites great places to sleep under the trees while leaving Northern Virginia's traffic jams behind.

After entering the park from Gunston Road, you'll turn right and follow the signs to reach the camping area. Once you reach the camp center and store, continue straight to reach sites 1–100 with hookups or go left for 101–150 sans electricity. Both spots offer flat sites in a nicely wooded area laden with pine, beech, and holly trees. Sites 31–38 form a small loop at the back of a much larger loop composed of the remaining sites with electricity. These encircle a grassy playing field and offer a considerable degree of privacy. Do not automatically eschew those sites with hookups because you wouldn't be using electricity. You might find them desirable if the park is busy. If you decide to go this route, try to get one of sites 31–38 located at the back on the small loop.

The sites without electric hookups are located a short distance away on the opposite side of the park's disc golf course and popular, large swimming pool. These are also laid out on a bigger and smaller loop in a more contained but heavily wooded area. Sites 101–150 appear smaller than

RATINGS

Beauty: ✿ ✿ ✿
Site privacy: ✿ ✿ ✿
Spaciousness: ✿ ✿ ✿
Quiet: ✿ ✿ ✿
Security: ✿ ✿ ✿
Cleanliness: ✿ ✿ ✿

MAP

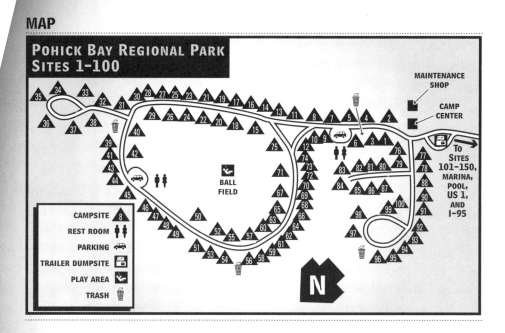

POHICK BAY REGIONAL PARK SITES 1–100

BALL FIELD

CAMPSITE
REST ROOM
PARKING
TRAILER DUMPSITE
PLAY AREA
TRASH

MAINTENANCE SHOP
CAMP CENTER

To SITES 101–150, MARINA, POOL, US 1, AND I-95

N

GETTING THERE

From I-95, take the Exit 163 (Lorton). Turn left onto Lorton Road, right onto US 1, and then left onto Gunston Road. Continue past the golf course to the park entrance on the left.

MAP

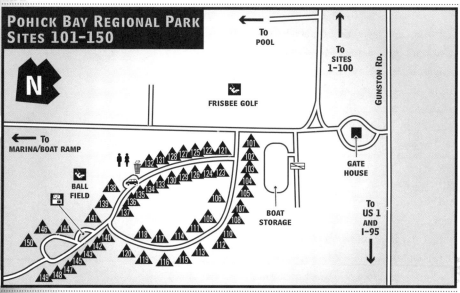

POHICK BAY REGIONAL PARK SITES 101–150

To POOL
To SITES 1–100
GUNSTON RD.

N

FRISBEE GOLF

To MARINA/BOAT RAMP

BALL FIELD

GATE HOUSE

BOAT STORAGE

To US 1 AND I-95

ADDRESS: Burke Lake Park
7315 Ox Road
Fairfax Station, VA
22039

OPERATED BY: Fairfax County Park
Authority

INFORMATION: (703) 323-6601

WEB SITE: www.co.fairfax.va.
us/parks/camp
grounds.htm

OPEN: Mid-April–October

SITES: 140

EACH SITE HAS: Picnic table and grill

ASSIGNMENT: First come, first
served

REGISTRATION: On site or by reservation

FACILITIES: Camp store, hot
showers, water, and
pay phone

PARKING: Limited to 1 camping vehicle and 1
non-camping vehicle

FEE: $20 per night for
first 4 people, $2 for
each extra person,
discounts for seniors

ELEVATION: 430 feet

RESTRICTIONS: Pets: Must be on
leash
Fires: Wood fires in
ring only; charcoal
fire in grill; wood
gathering prohibited
Alcohol: Prohibited
Vehicles: Up to 25
feet
Other: 7-day maxi-
mum stay; quiet time
10 p.m.–7 a.m.; all
campers must use a
camper, tent, or
other camping
device

room facilities. The wilderness area includes an ori-enteering course laid out for both beginners and advanced map and compass users.

The beauty of camping at Northern Virginia campgrounds like Burke Lake is not so much the ability to "rough it" but more the opportunity to sleep outdoors with all of the recreational, cultural, and educational activities that this vast suburb of Washington, D.C., has to offer. Don't think, how-ever, that you need to jump back into your vehicle to find something to do after setting up your camp-site. Therein lies the key to enjoying this facility managed by the Fairfax County Park Authority.

The lake itself offers a myriad of possibilities. Whether you bring your own canoe or rent a boat on site, you're sure to enjoy exploring Burke Lake's interesting coves as well as the waterfowl refuge on Vesper Island, which lies within its boundaries. Gasoline motors and sailboats are not allowed on the lake. Many Northern Virginian anglers come to the lake to cast a line for largemouth bass, walleye, muskie, catfish, crappie, perch, and bluegill. Bait and tackle are available at the park's marina or bring your own. Virginia fishing licenses are required.

Picnic areas with shelters for rent, an 18-hole, par-three golf course, driving range, Frisbee golf course, a miniature railroad, 5-mile walking trail, 18-station fitness trail, sand volleyball courts, playing fields, and even an ice cream parlor round out the kinds of activities that you'll find at this island of green amid the sprawling developments of Northern Virginia. There is no pool and swimming is not allowed in the lake. Don't let this discourage you, however, as campers wanting pools will head to Lake Fairfax or Pohick, leaving Burke Lake to you. It's enough to keep you having outdoor fun for days, but if you are camping at Burke Lake with the intent of touring the surrounding area, hop in the car for a

LAKE FAIRFAX PARK

> *Families with young'uns will find activities to enjoy during the summer at suburban Lake Fairfax Park.*

LAKE **FAIRFAX PARK'S** 476 wooded and open acres are tucked away in a unique, high-end planned community in the suburbs of Washington, D.C. Reston was conceived as a spacious urban area with a rural feel, complete with protected parks and greenery. Planners in the 1960s could never have predicted the high-tech boom that has flooded Northern Virginia with dense traffic and urban sprawl; nevertheless their foresight has preserved the forested environment that made Reston so desirable. Lake Fairfax is located near I-495, I-66, and VA 7, but you'd never know it as you drive down the wooded approach off Baron Cameron Avenue.

The first thing you'll notice as you enter the park is the Water Mine: Family Swimming Hole. Campers receive reduced rates into the attraction, which includes water slides, flumes, sprinklers, and floatables. You may scoff at this commercialism that obviously does not make for the ideal wilderness experience, but families with kids who are just breaking into camping will find that the Water Mine makes the experience a lot more palatable for the youngsters. And in the summer, most of us will find the water attraction downright refreshing since swimming has not been allowed in the lake for several years.

Driving into the park, you'll notice a more natural environment with tree-lined streams alongside the road, which climbs to the hilltop campground. You will also pass signs for the requisite ball fields as in any other Northern Virginia municipal park. In addition, Lake Fairfax Park offers a cricket field—a

RATINGS

Beauty: ✿ ✿ ✿
Site privacy: ✿ ✿ ✿
Spaciousness: ✿ ✿ ✿
Quiet: ✿ ✿ ✿
Security: ✿ ✿ ✿
Cleanliness: ✿ ✿ ✿

MAP

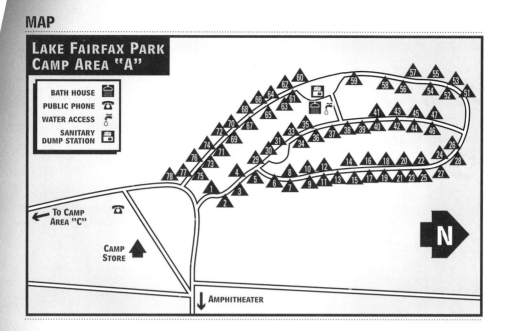

LAKE FAIRFAX PARK CAMP AREA "A"

BATH HOUSE
PUBLIC PHONE
WATER ACCESS
SANITARY DUMP STATION

To Camp Area "C"

CAMP STORE

AMPHITHEATER

N

GETTING THERE

From the I-495 Beltway, take Exit 47A west for 6.5 miles. Turn left onto Baron Cameron Avenue (SR 606) and then left onto Lake Fairfax Drive. The park entrance is a short distance ahead.

outdoor experience than most others in this guide. But this is Northern Virginia, and many families with children will find a lot to enjoy during the summer at Lake Fairfax Park.

KEY INFORMATION

ADDRESS: Bull Run Regional Park
7700 Bull Run Drive
Centreville, VA
20121

OPERATED BY: Northern Virginia Regional Park Authority

INFORMATION: (703) 631-0550

WEB SITE: www.nvrpa.org/ bullrunpark

OPEN: Mid-March–mid-October

SITES: 150

EACH SITE HAS: Picnic table, grill, campfire ring

ASSIGNMENT: First come, first served

REGISTRATION: By reservation or on arrival

FACILITIES: Camp store, laundry, hot showers, pay phone, and water

PARKING: At campsites; max 2 vehicles per site

FEE: $16; $19.50 with electric up to 4 campers; additional $2.50 per person, limit 7; discounts for regional residents

ELEVATION: 160 feet

RESTRICTIONS: Pets: Must be attended and on leash
Fires: Wood fires only within ground ring; only charcoal in grills; all fires must be attended; no collecting downed wood
Alcohol: Prohibited
Vehicles: Up to 45 feet
Other: Quiet hours 10 p.m.–7 a.m.; maximum stay of 7 consecutive days

gain access to this fascinating piece of U.S. and Virginia Civil War history.

Be sure to stop in the town of Manassas, especially at the visitor center located in the newly renovated train depot. A fascinating walking or driving tour of Old Town Manassas starts at the depot. In this designated Main Street Community, you'll find a wide selection of fine restaurants, art studios, galleries, and antique shops, as well as the Manassas Volunteer Fire Company Museum. For day tours to Washington, D.C., leave your car in Manassas and catch a train. Request a parking permit from the visitor center or leave from Manassas Park, where there are 677 spaces.

By the time you approach Bull Run Regional Park's entrance, the drone of I-66 will have wafted off into the background. Drive 2 more miles to reach the campground and you'll get an idea of the park's other offerings, including picnic shelters, miniature and Frisbee golf courses, soccer fields, a large swimming pool, a wildlife-viewing bench by a waterhole, and a shooting center featuring skeet, archery, and a sporting clay course. The expansive, grassy playing fields and sycamore trees on the park's 1,500 flat acres bordering Cub Run and Bull Run suggest a flood plain—but the campground is located on higher ground with its own emergency access, so high water is generally not a problem.

The heavily wooded campground is located near the center of the park. Sites are well spaced, private, flat, and spread out along a large loop with three smaller inner loops. A third of the 150 sites are nonelectric; these are located along the outer edge of the campground loop. While campers may have particular preferences on arrival, the combination of dense oak woods, understory, and ample size and spacing of campsites is such that you'll have a hard time finding fault with any of the nonelectric sites. Municipal parks must be many things to many

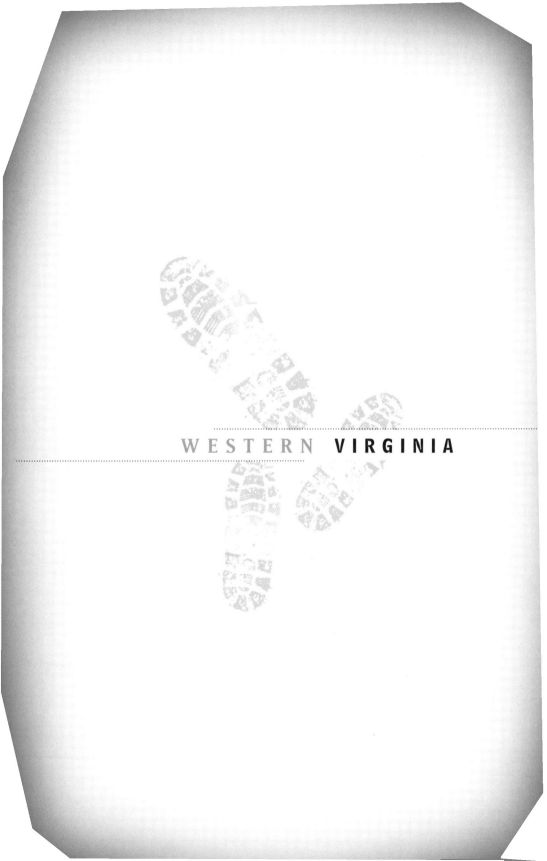

WESTERN **VIRGINIA**

ADDRESS: Mathews Arm
Campground
Shenandoah
National Park
3655 US 211 East
Luray, VA
22835-9036

OPERATED BY: National Park
Service

INFORMATION: (540) 999-3500

WEB SITE: www.nps.gov/shen

OPEN: Weather-dependent;
spring–October

SITES: 179

EACH SITE HAS: Picnic table and fire
grill

ASSIGNMENT: First come, first
served

REGISTRATION: On arrival

FACILITIES: Flush toilets

PARKING: At campsite and
near amphitheater

FEE: $16 per night plus
$10 park entrance

ELEVATION: 2,800 feet

RESTRICTIONS: Pets: Must be
attended and on
leash shorter than 6
feet; clean up after
pet
Fires: Only in camp-
stoves and fireplaces
Alcohol: Permitted
Vehicles: No limit
Other: Do not carve,
chop, or damage any
trees; wash dishes at
campsite, not at rest
rooms, but gray
water must be dis-
posed of in service
sinks at rest rooms;
campsite capacity is
6 people, 2 tents, 2
vehicles per site;
quiet hours
10 p.m.–6 a.m.

and C. Privacy is provided by mature oak and hickory trees as well as the numerous rock out-crops that punctuate the area. Despite the uneven slope over much of Mathews Arm Campground, campsites are level; you'll have no trouble pitching your tent. Those sites closest to the entrance station are more open and will attract RVers despite the lack of RV hookups. While there are many desirable sites throughout the campground, most are adjacent to one of the loop roads. At the back of the campground, however, is the "Tents Only" area comprised of walk-in sites B89–B102, which are set apart. You'll have to carry your gear a short distance from the central parking area, but the quiet and privacy make it well worth the minor extra effort.

Opportunities for hiking abound with 101 miles of the 2,100-mile Appalachian Trail running through the park. Many thru-hikers agree that the section of Appalachian Trail through Shenandoah National Park is the most beautiful of the trail's entire length from Georgia to Maine. Shenandoah also includes more than 400 additional miles of trails, most of which connect to the Appalachian Trail. Bicycling is popular on paved Skyline Drive but bikes are pro-hibited on trails within the park.

A population of some 6,000 white-tailed deer resides within the park's boundaries, and you're sure to encounter them at some time during your visit. Keep in mind, however, that it is illegal to feed park animals. An estimated 300–600 black bears also live within Shenandoah National Park. Seriously heed park warnings to store your food in bear-proof con-tainers, keep food out of your tent and at least 100 yards away, and use park-provided, bear-proof food-storage poles or suspend food from trees at least ten feet from the ground and four feet from either tree. The tents-only area at Mathews Arm Campground features several food-storage poles.

BIG MEADOWS CAMPGROUND

> *You're likely to see song sparrows, meadowlarks, grouse, foxes, and skunks.*

BIG MEADOWS is Shenandoah National Park's largest treeless area, encompassing a barren plateau that is approximately 640 acres. It's believed that Native Americans cleared the area to create favorable grazing conditions. European settlers overgrazed this site with beef cattle, especially during the Civil War. Park officials have waged an ongoing battle against the growth of black locust and blackberry that would, if left unchecked, take over the meadow. In the past, Park Service officials used combinations of burning and mowing to hold back the growth of invasive vegetation, but eventually realized that the burning actually helped the black locust and blackberry spread. New strategies have aided in the establishment of meadow grasses. Today the dominant shrub growth in the meadow is blueberry with swamp varieties such as marsh marigold, swamp fern, and Canadian burnet growing in wetter areas with some 270 species of vascular plants. In addition to the white-tailed deer that wander seemingly carefree through the meadow, you're also likely to see song sparrows, meadowlarks, grouse, foxes, and skunks.

The park's dedication was held at Big Meadows, the spiritual center of Skyline Drive, on July 3, 1936. President Franklin D. Roosevelt himself was on hand to formally open the facilities at Shenandoah National Park. The meadow is located across Skyline Drive from the Harry F. Byrd Visitor Center, which houses informative exhibits, a library, an auditorium, interpretive programs, and an array of literature pertaining to Shenandoah National Park that is on sale in the small gift shop.

RATINGS

Beauty: ✿ ✿ ✿ ✿
Site privacy: ✿ ✿ ✿ ✿
Spaciousness: ✿ ✿ ✿ ✿
Quiet: ✿ ✿ ✿ ✿
Security: ✿ ✿ ✿ ✿
Cleanliness: ✿ ✿ ✿ ✿ ✿

MAP

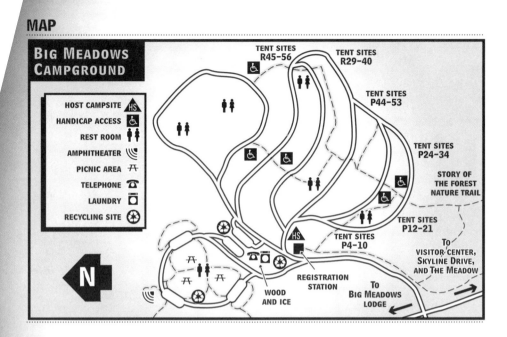

Big Meadows Campground

- HOST CAMPSITE — HS
- HANDICAP ACCESS
- REST ROOM
- AMPHITHEATER
- PICNIC AREA
- TELEPHONE
- LAUNDRY
- RECYCLING SITE

TENT SITES R45–56

TENT SITES R29–40

TENT SITES P44–53

TENT SITES P24–34

STORY OF THE FOREST NATURE TRAIL

TENT SITES P12–21

To VISITOR CENTER, SKYLINE DRIVE, AND THE MEADOW

TENT SITES P4–10

REGISTRATION STATION

WOOD AND ICE

To BIG MEADOWS LODGE

N

GETTING THERE

From the Swift Run Gap Entrance Station at mile 65.7, drive north on Skyline Drive to Big Meadows at mile 51.2.

Nature Trail is a relatively easy walk starting from the Byrd Visitor Center. Interpretive signs explain various aspects of the surrounding forest. The 3.3-mile Lewis Falls Trail provides more of a challenge in terms of length and change in elevation after it exits from the amphitheater parking lot. The hike to the 81-foot falls is worth the effort.

Camp Hoover (aka Rapidan Camp), located across from Big Meadows 6.3 miles down the Rapidan Fire Road, was a favorite getaway for President Herbert Hoover. The walk to Camp Hoover can be shortened to a 4-mile out-and-back by taking the Mill Prong Trail. Camp Hoover is a beautiful spot where 3 of the original 13 cabins remain at the confluence of Mill Prong, Laurel Prong, and the Rapidan River. In the summer, three-hour van tours are available several days a week. Sign up in advance at the Byrd Visitor Center.

ADDRESS: Lewis Mountain Campground 3655 US 211 East Luray, VA 22835-9036

OPERATED BY: National Park Service

INFORMATION: (540) 999-3500

WEB SITE: www.nps.gov/shen

OPEN: Weather-dependent; early spring to late autumn

SITES: 32

EACH SITE HAS: Picnic table and fire grill

ASSIGNMENT: Campers can choose from available sites

REGISTRATION: On arrival

FACILITIES: Camp store, laundry, coin-operated show-ers, and flush toilets

PARKING: At campsite and next to camp store

FEE: $16 in addition to $10 park entrance

ELEVATION: 3,396 feet

RESTRICTIONS: Pets: Must be attended and on leash shorter than 6 feet; clean up after pet
Fires: Only in camp-stoves and fireplaces
Alcohol: Permitted
Vehicles: Up to 30 feet on pull-through sites
Other: Do not dam-age any trees; wash dishes at campsite, not at rest rooms, but gray water must be disposed of in service sinks at rest rooms; campsite capacity is 6 people, 2 tents, 2 vehicles per site; quiet hours 10 p.m.–6 a.m.

cially important not to eat or store food in your tent lest you have unwanted late-night visitors of the large and furry kind.

This campground doesn't offer access to an abundance of hiking trails as do the park's other campgrounds. However, nowhere in Shenandoah National Park are you too far from the more than 500 miles of trails that crisscross the 196,000-acre park. The half-mile (point-to-point) Lewis Moun-tain East Trail departs from site 16 on its short ascent to Lewis Mountain via a mossy and fern-lined path. Numerous other hikes are accessible via the Appalachian Trail, which you can reach from site 3. Just as the 105-mile Skyline Drive forms the park's backbone for driving, 101 miles of the Appalachian Trail form a spine of sorts for hikers. Shenandoah's abundant side trails are just a short drive away.

Either by walking south along the Appalachian Trail or driving on Skyline Drive to milepost 59.5, you can reach the start of the Pocosin Mission Trail. You'll pass one of the Potomac Appalachian Trail Cabins as you amble along the fire road to the site of an old Episcopal mission, established around 1904, complete with a fascinating, overgrown ceme-tery. Turn around and head back for a pretty, easy 1.9-mile walk in the woods. Stretch this into a longer and more challenging 5.6-mile out-and-back by continuing on the yellow-blazed trail to Pocosin Hollow before returning.

Head north a short distance to milepost 56.4 to get onto the Bearfence Mountain Trail. You'll do your share of huffing and puffing as you scramble over the volcanic boulders, but by the time you reach the 3,640-foot summit of Bearfence Mountain, you'll enjoy a panoramic view that on a clear day will seem to go on forever. Backtrack or loop around for a 1.2-mile outing. Be sure to pick up one of the trail guides to Shenandoah Park that is listed

LOFT MOUNTAIN CAMPGROUND

> *Enjoy great panoramic views of the neighboring peaks, valley, and piedmont from this 3,400-foot perch.*

LOFT MOUNTAIN CAMPGROUND is located just off Skyline Drive in the southern section of Shenandoah National Park at mile 79.5. It is unique among the park's other campgrounds in that it is located at the top of Big Flat Mountain. As a result, there are great east and west panoramic views of the neighboring peaks, valley, and piedmont from this 3,400-foot perch. Another unusual feature at Loft Mountain Campground is the absence of mature, lofty hardwood trees that populate most of Shenandoah National Park. This mountaintop was once pastureland, so instead of trees there is an abundance of thick, low-growing shrubbery. This offers a considerable degree of privacy between campsites, and the dense vegetation diminishes the feeling of being crowded at Skyline Drive's largest campground, which contains 219 sites. Loft Mountain Campground is the southernmost of Shenandoah's campgrounds and is the ideal base from which to explore this end of the National Park.

The campground consists of Loop A, which circumscribes the entire campground with smaller loops B through H cutting across the center of Loop A. Most of the sites are private and spacious, but those who want to completely avoid RVs and enjoy the feeling of being off by themselves should look at the 54 walk-in tent sites located on the outer edge of Loop A. Parking is nearby with one space reserved for each site, but you'll have to carry your gear a short distance to your home in the woods which includes a picnic table, grill, and tent pad.

Fall weekends are the most popular times for camping here as well as in the rest of Shenandoah

RATINGS

Beauty: ✿ ✿ ✿ ✿
Site privacy: ✿ ✿ ✿ ✿
Spaciousness: ✿ ✿ ✿ ✿
Quiet: ✿ ✿ ✿ ✿
Security: ✿ ✿ ✿ ✿
Cleanliness: ✿ ✿ ✿ ✿ ✿

MAP

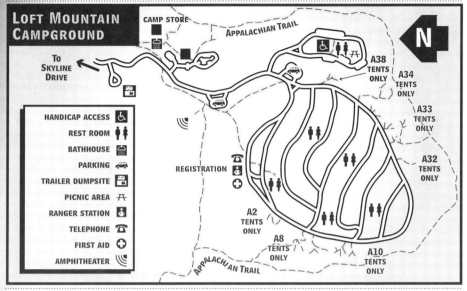

LOFT MOUNTAIN CAMPGROUND

CAMP STORE
APPALACHIAN TRAIL

To SKYLINE DRIVE

N

A38 TENTS ONLY
A34 TENTS ONLY
A33 TENTS ONLY
A32 TENTS ONLY

REGISTRATION

A2 TENTS ONLY
A8 TENTS ONLY
A10 TENTS ONLY

APPALACHIAN TRAIL

HANDICAP ACCESS
REST ROOM
BATHHOUSE
PARKING
TRAILER DUMPSITE
PICNIC AREA
RANGER STATION
TELEPHONE
FIRST AID
AMPHITHEATER

GETTING THERE

From the Swift Run Gap Entrance Station at mile 65.7, drive south on Skyline Drive to the campground entrance at mile 79.5.

you to a 3,290-foot perch on the side of Loft Mountain for some equally awesome views. On a clear day, you can see west to Massanutten Mountain.

ADDRESS: Sky Meadows State
Park Campground
11012 Edmonds Lane
Delaplane, VA 20144

OPERATED BY: Virginia State
Department of
Conservation and
Recreation

INFORMATION: (540) 592-3556

WEB SITE: www.dcr.state.va.us/
parks

OPEN: Year-round, weather
permitting

SITES: 12

EACH SITE HAS: Picnic table, fire ring

ASSIGNMENT: Reserve or on
arrival

REGISTRATION: Reservations
through (800) 933-
PARK or on arrival

FACILITIES: Hand pump and
vault toilets

PARKING: Central parking
area, walk to all
sites; 1 car included,
additional cars $3
per night

FEE: $9 per night; $3 per
additional dog

ELEVATION: 1,000 feet

RESTRICTIONS: Pets: Must be on
leash shorter than 6
feet
Fires: Only in camp-
stoves and fireplaces
Alcohol: Prohibited
Vehicles: None, must
park in central park-
ing area
Other: Tents only;
campers must arrive
before dusk.

oped scenic area. Additional parcels of land were added later, bringing the total acreage to 1,862 acres, but Sky Meadows has continued to respect Mellon's request. Aside from the central parking lot and visitor center area, there is only a picnic area, fishing pond, campground, and trails.

The visitor center building was not added to the park, but is an existing 150-year-old structure. Mount Bleak House has been authentically furnished as a Civil War–era farmhouse, and is being restored and interpreted as the Abner Settle family home. The Settle family lived in Mount Bleak around 1860 and sold the property around 1868. It was purchased in 1870 by George M. Slater, one of Mosby's Rangers during the Civil War. The land changed hands several times before being rescued from development by Paul Mellon. Mount Bleak House is open all week during the summer and on spring and fall weekends. Tours are offered on weekends and holidays, with interpretive programs taking place behind it in the summer.

Sky Meadows has two loop bridle trails and 10 miles of hiking trails, in addition to Appalachian Trail access. Gap Run Trail is a 1.2-mile trail that begins at the edge of the visitor center parking lot and passes through the campground before continuing on to meet the 1.7-mile North Ridge Trail. A right turn takes hikers back to the parking lot, or to the 0.7-mile Piedmont Overlook Trail. A left turn takes hikers up the ridge to the famed Appalachian Trail. The 1.6-mile South Ridge Trail offers the option of returning to the Gap Run Trail by a different route. The park is a three-day Appalachian Trail hike from Harpers Ferry, West Virginia. Cars can be left in the parking lot for this time as long as the daily fee is paid and the camping permit is displayed with the words "AT Hiker" written on it.

Were it not for Northern Virginia's legendary rush-hour traffic, Sky Meadows would be just an

ELIZABETH FURNACE
RECREATION AREA

> *Fort Valley's natural camouflage has protected its inhabitants from development.*

THE ELIZABETH FURNACE RECREATION AREA is nestled in Fort Valley, a 22-mile long valley hidden at the northern end of the 50-mile long Massanutten Mountain. You can easily drive right by Fort Valley without noticing it's there, and its elusiveness and inaccessibility has been exploited throughout history. In the 1700s, an English miner named Powell counterfeited coins from Fort Valley's ore, and vanished into Fort Valley any time authorities tried to capture him. The locals referred to the area as "Powell's Fort Valley." George Washington is said to have considered it both as an alternative to the winter camp at Valley Forge, and as a last-resort bunker if things had gone badly during the Revolutionary War.

Fort Valley's natural camouflage has protected its inhabitants not just from invading armies but also from development. You won't find a Wal-Mart or McDonald's in Fort Valley, and residents often must drive as much as 30 miles to get to a major supermarket. The valley is covered in undeveloped, green National Forest and farmland. Many of the original roads and trails were constructed by the CCC before World War II.

Today Fort Valley is clearly marked on all Virginia maps and SR 678 goes into the valley from Strasburg, so the campground is accessible from both urban Northern Virginia and Washington, D.C. The trails of Fort Valley and densely wooded campsites of Elizabeth Furnace get more than their share of use.

Access to this campground can be restricted after times of heavy rain when the creek overflows its banks. Under average conditions, however, it provides a nice backdrop to this quiet campground

RATINGS

Beauty: ☆ ☆ ☆
Site privacy: ☆ ☆ ☆
Spaciousness: ☆ ☆ ☆
Quiet: ☆ ☆ ☆
Security: ☆ ☆ ☆
Cleanliness: ☆ ☆ ☆

MAP

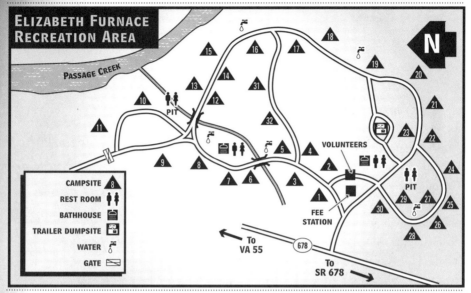

ELIZABETH FURNACE RECREATION AREA

PASSAGE CREEK

N

VOLUNTEERS

PIT

FEE STATION

CAMPSITE	8
REST ROOM	👫
BATHHOUSE	🏠
TRAILER DUMPSITE	🖶
WATER	🚰
GATE	▱

To VA 55

678

To SR 678

GETTING THERE

From I-81 Exit 296, follow VA 55 east through Strasburg. After 6.5 miles, turn right onto SR 678. Go 3.5 miles to the campground entrance on the left.

pared to yield the right-of-way to hikers who frequent the area, especially on weekends.

The yellow-blazed, 4.5-mile (point-to-point) Signal Knob Trail is a popular trail skirting the northern end of Massanutten. It offers some outstanding views including those from Buzzard Rock Overlook and Fort Valley Overlook. To avoid a 9-mile out-and-back hike, plan to return via the Massanutten Mountain West and Bear Wallow Trails. A particularly picturesque spot is Mudhole Gap through which Little Passage Creek passes between the Massanutten West Trail and the Little Sluice forest road.

A popular time to visit the area is in September during the Elizabeth Furnace Folkways Festival, when traditional artisans demonstrate basket making, woodcarving, weaving, and blacksmithing. Anglers will definitely want to bring their gear and do some fishing in the trout-stocked Passage Creek that runs through this Recreation Area along SR 678. Fall-color season is also popular, when the leaves of Fort Valley take center stage.

ADDRESS: Raymond R. "Andy" Guest Jr. Shenandoah River State Park Daughter of Stars Drive P.O. Box 235 Bentonville, VA 22610

OPERATED BY: Virginia State Department of Conservation and Recreation

INFORMATION: (540) 622-6840

WEB SITE: www.dcr.state.va.us/parks

OPEN: Year-round, weather permitting

SITES: 10

EACH SITE HAS: Picnic table, fire grill, lantern pole

ASSIGNMENT: First come, first served

REGISTRATION: Reserve through (800) 933-PARK at www.reserveamerica.com or on arrival

FACILITIES: Water, hot showers, dish sink, flush and vault toilets, wagons, and canoe launch

PARKING: Central parking area

FEE: $18 per night

ELEVATION: 600 feet

RESTRICTIONS: Pets: On leash; clean up after pet
Fires: Only in campstoves and fireplaces
Alcohol: Prohibited
Vehicles: None at sites, walk-in only
Other: Use trash bins at "Three Bends Overlook"; use designated river access points; no cutting of live vegetation; quiet hours 10 p.m.–8 a.m.

mile marker 32, 4 miles downstream from a low-water bridge.

Tent pads are palatial by comparison to similar sites throughout the region, and sites are widely spaced with riparian buffers to provide privacy. Four sites are directly on the riverfront, but the sites set further back in the forest are scenic and secluded. A new bathhouse with running water, showers, and a utility sink was added to River Right Campground in 2003, making these ten coveted sites even more desirable. Reservations are a must at this small campground but individual sites cannot be booked; you must choose from available sites. Canoe or walk in early.

Canoes cannot be rented at the park itself, but plenty of nearby commercial outfitters supply canoes. The National Forest Service runs nine primitive canoe-in campsites along the Shenandoah River for those who want to rough it. Sites are strictly "leave no trace" and are located at mile markers 6, 8–9, 12–14.5, 16–19, and 24–25. The contact station can also recommend several nearby private campgrounds if the ten Shenandoah River sites are full. Canoe novices needing handholding might consider one of the 25 shady tent-only campsites on South Page Valley Road near Luray at Shenandoah River Outfitters (phone (540) 743-4159), a private company that rents canoes, kayaks, and inner tubes. Commercial tent-only campgrounds are rare, and while not as nice as the pristine new Shenandoah River State Park campground, this one features a pleasant wooded grove with fire rings, picnic tables, and bathhouse, along with canoe rental.

Once you're done canoeing, there are plenty of options available. Shenandoah National Park and Fort Valley are both nearby, as are the towns of Luray and Front Royal. Thirteen miles of trails crisscross Shenandoah River State Park, of which

CAMP ROOSEVELT RECREATION AREA

> *You'd be hard-pressed to find quieter and larger campsites anywhere.*

THE SINGLE GREATEST conservation movement in history began on March 9, 1933, when President Franklin D. Roosevelt created the Civilian Conservation Corps in response to the Great Depression. The goal was twofold: to put the nation's young men back to work and to conserve forests and natural environments.

A month later, the first troop of "Roosevelt's Boys" marched into the George Washington National Forest and broke ground on the inaugural CCC camp—Camp Roosevelt. FDR's "Army With Shovels" went on to plant two billion trees and build roads, bridges, trails, and 800 state parks. The results of their work can be admired throughout the country, but locally CCC work endures along Skyline Drive, Fort Valley, and throughout National Parks and forests. By the time World War II arrived, three million men were ardent conservationists.

It is fitting, then, that the campground at Camp Roosevelt is peaceful, undeveloped, and wooded. The ten campsites are spacious with plenty of vegetation and land between them. You'd be hard-pressed to find quieter and larger campsites anywhere.

Camp Roosevelt is located a short distance from the Massanutten Visitor Center on US 211, on Massanutten Mountain at the lower end of Fort Valley. The entrance to the recreation area is at the intersection of FDR 274 and SR 675, with the picnic area straight ahead and the campground to the left. The campground loop is arranged around a grassy central area where the bathhouse is located, and the entire site is right on top of the old CCC barracks and recreation hall. Adjacent to the campground is

RATINGS

Beauty: ✿ ✿ ✿
Site privacy: ✿ ✿ ✿ ✿
Spaciousness: ✿ ✿ ✿ ✿
Quiet: ✿ ✿ ✿
Security: ✿ ✿ ✿
Cleanliness: ✿ ✿ ✿

MAP

CAMP ROOSEVELT RECREATION AREA

To EDINBURG

To LURRAY

675

To PICNIC AREA

N

REGISTRATION

CAMPSITE
REST ROOM
BATHHOUSE
PICNIC AREA

GETTING THERE

From Luray, follow SR 675 for 9 miles to the campground entrance.

Forest. Additionally, nearby Luray features caverns, canoeing, and plenty of attractions for kids. Shenandoah Caverns and the New Market Battlefield, site of an 1864 Civil War battle in which 250 cadets from Virginia Military Institute successfully fought, are both nearby off of US 11, or you can go further up into the mountains to explore Skyline Drive.

ADDRESS: Hone Quarry
Recreation Area
Dry River Ranger
District
401 Oakwood Dr.
Harrisonburg, VA
22801

OPERATED BY: U.S. Forest Service

INFORMATION: (540) 432-0187

WEB SITE: www.southern
region.fs.fed.us/gwj

OPEN: Year-round; snow
and ice may restrict
winter use

SITES: 10

EACH SITE HAS: Fireplace grill, picnic table, lantern
pole

ASSIGNMENT: Camper can choose
from available sites

REGISTRATION: On arrival

FACILITIES: Vault toilets and well
with hand pump

PARKING: At campsite and picnic area

FEE: $5 per night

ELEVATION: 1,880 feet

RESTRICTIONS: Pets: On leash only
Fires: In fire rings,
stoves, or grills only
Alcohol: Prohibited
Vehicles: Up to 21
feet
Other: Do not carve,
chop, or damage any
live trees; keep noise
at a reasonable
level; non-gasoline-
powered boats only
allowed in quarry;
quiet time 10 p.m.–
6 a.m.

Swimming is prohibited. For alternate fishing desti-
nations, Hearthstone Lake is just 7 miles away on
FDR 101, and Switzer Lake is just north of here in
the shadow of High Knob on US 33. For those who
enjoy their trout fishing from closer banks, Hone
Quarry Run is an option, as well as Briery Branch
Lake. Those looking to take a swim in the National
Forest will find the Todd Lake Recreation Area,
some 12.5 miles south of Hone Quarry, to be an
inviting destination.

For spectacular views into West Virginia and
across the Shenandoah Valley, leave the campground and turn right onto SR 924. Keep climbing
Shenandoah Mountain until you reach the crest of
Reddish Knob. Don't be surprised if you see some
intrepid bicyclists attempting the assault on Reddish
Knob. You'll find parking as well as an incredible
panorama from this 4,397-foot perch.

This section of the National Forest is popular
among Harrisonburg's large number of mountain
bikers, and many of the more desirable trails and
woods roads funnel down off of Shenandoah Mountain and converge on Hone Quarry. Mud Pond
Gap, Slate Springs Trail, and California Ridge are
but a few of the local, well-used trails within a short
distance of the Hone Quarry campground. This is a
great area for hikers and equestrians; but be prepared to share the trail whether you're on two legs
or two wheels.

FDR 62 becomes increasingly rocky as it
climbs Shenandoah Mountain toward Flagpole
Knob. Along the way the rough road ends where
Mines Run Trail begins before merging into the
Slate Springs Trails. If you're planning to do any
exploring up here, pick up a National Forest map of
the Dry River District. Hone Quarry is set among
an incredible network of trails, and these inexpensive maps will give you an idea of the trails that surround your campsite. Undoubtedly you'll find, as I

TODD LAKE
RECREATION AREA

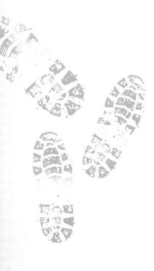

> *Camping at Todd Lake will open up a world of outdoor activities.*

LIVING JUST A HALF-HOUR'S drive from Todd Lake over the course of my 20 years as a Shenandoah Valley resident, I confess to having spent more time at this recreation area taking a dip in the 7.5-acre lake after a rigorous mountain bike ride or a day-long family outing than as an overnight camper. No matter how far away you live, however, you'll find that camping at Todd Lake opens up a world of outdoor activities in this part of the George Washington and Jefferson National Forests. Forest Service representatives suggest that campers looking for optimal seclusion at this or any other National Forest campground should plan their visit during mid-week or outside of the busy summer months.

This recreation area is located south-west of Harrisonburg. After a short ride through some of the Shenandoah Valley's most endearing back roads, you'll enter the Todd Lake Recreation Area from FDR 95, where the road turns from hard surface to gravel. The campground sits on a knoll to the left of the main road, with the day-use area straight ahead just inside the gated entrance. After a short downhill, you'll see the large parking area for the lake on the right. Continue past here for access to the recreation area's expansive wooded picnic area that ends at the edge of the lake. There's a roped-off sand beach and swimming area, and the additional lake area is available for anglers and non-motorized boats. Boaters and anglers looking for a little more elbowroom will, however, drive a few miles to the larger Elkhorn Lake.

Half of Todd Lake's 20 campsites (1–4, 16–20) are spaced along the straight part of the camp road

RATINGS

Beauty: ✿ ✿ ✿ ✿
Site privacy: ✿ ✿ ✿
Spaciousness: ✿ ✿ ✿ ✿ ✿
Quiet: ✿ ✿ ✿
Security: ✿ ✿ ✿
Cleanliness: ✿ ✿ ✿ ✿

MAP

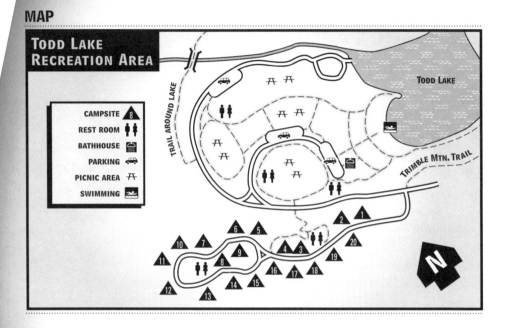

TODD LAKE RECREATION AREA

TODD LAKE

TRAIL AROUND LAKE

TRIMBLE MTN. TRAIL

CAMPSITE	8
REST ROOM	👫
BATHHOUSE	🏠
PARKING	🚗
PICNIC AREA	🏕
SWIMMING	🏊

N

GETTING THERE

From Bridgewater, follow VA 42 for 3 miles south to Mossy Creek. Continue on SR 747 where VA 42 bends sharply to the left. Take SR 731 for 1 mile before turning left onto SR 730. Go 3 miles and turn right onto SR 718. Follow this for a mile until it turns into FDR 95. Continue on FDR 95 for 2 miles to the entrance to Todd Lake.

Mountain's relatively gentle slopes before crossing a steeper and rockier Lookout Mountain.

Area mountain biking opportunities are unlimited if you combine existing trails and Forest Service roads. I've long enjoyed the 14-mile Great Lakes Loop that passes Todd Lake on gravel roads. Start from Todd Lake, heading uphill on FDR 95A before circling back on FDR 95 along a series of challenging ascents and exhilarating descents that take you past Elkhorn Lake and the Staunton Dam.

KEY INFORMATION

ADDRESS: Sherando Lake
Recreation Area
Glenwood and Ped-
lar Ranger Districts
P.O. Box 10
Natural Bridge
Station, VA 24579

OPERATED BY: U.S. Forest Service

INFORMATION: (540) 291-2188

WEB SITE: www.southern
region.fs.fed.us/gwj

OPEN: April 1–end of
October

SITES: 65

EACH SITE HAS: Picnic table, fire
grill, lantern pole

ASSIGNMENT: Your choice

REGISTRATION: On arrival

FACILITIES: Water, flush toilets,
hot showers in B and
C loops and in lake
bathhouse, drink
machines

PARKING: At campsites, picnic
area, and lake

FEE: $15 per night; $20
per night with
hookups

ELEVATION: 1,860 feet

RESTRICTIONS: Pets: On leash and
attended at all times;
not allowed on
beach or in swim-
ming areas
Fires: Camp stoves
and grills only; must
be attended.
Alcohol: Permitted at
campsite only.
Vehicles: No limit at
Loop B and Loop C
Campgrounds
Other: Quiet hours
10 p.m.–6 a.m.;
length of stay is lim-
ited to 21 consecu-
tive days; swimming
and picnic areas
close at dark.

renovated, but you'll still find some of the original stonework from the park's construction by CCC workers in the 1930s. To really admire their accomplishments at Sherando, take a close look at the stone beachfront bathhouse and pavilion.

The Riverbend Campground, aka Campground B, lies along the South River (actually a creek) that runs through this recreation area. It is flat, open, and the only loop that has hookups for RVs. A little farther down the road is the Meadow Loop, or Campground C, with 18 sites that are flat, open and lack hookups.

There are actually two lakes at Sherando. The seven-acre Upper Sherando Lake, near the end of the main park road, was created by the Soil Conservation Service in the 1960s and is designated for fishing. The 25-acre lower lake has an attractive swimming beach with a roped-off wading area. Stronger swimmers can practice their strokes on the way out to an island that is approximately a quarter-mile from the beach. Anglers can cast their line anywhere along the shore away from the beach, although many choose to do so at the lower end of the lake by the dam. The lakeside trail will take you there as will a turnoff from the camp road 1 mile after the entrance station.

Hikers and mountain bikers will find much to do at Sherando Lake, as they explore trails that meander as well as those that climb up the surrounding mountains to the famed Blue Ridge Parkway. After passing site 5 on Campground A loop, you'll notice the well-blazed Blue Loop Trail, which goes 0.5 mile to Lookout Rock and connects with other trails for longer and more strenuous climbs, including a 4-mile ascent (one way) to Bald Mountain. The White Rock Gap Trail is a favorite among mountain bikers as a way to ascend and descend to and from the Blue Ridge Parkway. So whether you're looking for a little quiet time in the woods or

NORTH CREEK CAMPGROUND

> *This no-frills area is shadowed by towering hemlocks and even more towering mountain ridges.*

NORTH CREEK CAMPGROUND lies secluded at the foot of the Blue Ridge Mountains. It is a no-frills area where you can pitch a tent in the shadow of towering hemlocks and even more towering mountain ridges with few other campers around. There is no bathhouse, just vault toilets and water pumps, but camping at North Creek is several steps above backpacking. You can drive to your site along a fast-moving trout stream and find a grill on which to cook your catch of the day or something from your cooler, with a picnic table on which to eat or just sit. Additionally, there is a garbage bin, dump station, and helpful volunteer campground host. North Creek Campground is not representative of all the campgrounds in this guide, but in many ways its scenic location and relatively primitive facilities connote the essence of what *The Best in Tent Camping* is all about. Not everyone is looking for this kind of back-to-nature experience, nor is it readily accessible to most people. And so this book contains a sampling of camping experiences with a variety of amenities and, ideally, something for everybody.

The campground is bordered by North Creek, a stocked trout stream that completely encircles this spartan 15-site facility en route to the James River, which is located just west of here. All of these insular sites lie on a single gravel loop along the creek in an area of dense pine and hemlock trees with understory vegetation that allows for separation between sites. The better-than-average size of the sites combined with the privacy from others means that campers are likely to find ample seclusion here.

RATINGS

Beauty: ✿ ✿ ✿ ✿
Site privacy: ✿ ✿ ✿ ✿
Spaciousness: ✿ ✿ ✿
Quiet: ✿ ✿ ✿
Security: ✿ ✿
Cleanliness: ✿ ✿ ✿

MAP

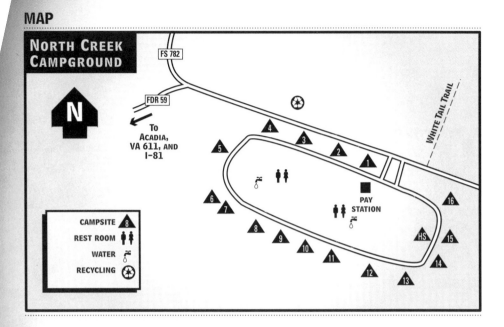

NORTH CREEK CAMPGROUND

FS 782

FDR 59

N

To ACADIA, VA 611, AND I-81

WHITE TAIL TRAIL

PAY STATION

CAMPSITE 8
REST ROOM 👫
WATER 🚰
RECYCLING ♻

GETTING THERE

From I-81, take Exit 168 onto SR 614. Follow SR 614 for 3 miles before turning left onto FDR 59. Continue for 2.5 miles to North Creek Campground.

Whether you come here for outdoor challenges or quiet respite, you're sure to get your batteries recharged after a few days at North Creek.

ADDRESS: Otter Creek
Campground
Blue Ridge Parkway
199 Hemphill Knob
Road
Asheville, NC 28803

OPERATED BY: National Park
Service

INFORMATION: (434) 299-5941

WEB SITE: www.nps.gov/blri

OPEN: May 1–October 31;
occasional reduced-
fee, reduced-service
winter camping
available

SITES: 45

EACH SITE HAS: Picnic table, fire
ring, lantern pole

ASSIGNMENT: First come, first
served

REGISTRATION: Self-registration
on-site

FACILITIES: Restaurant, water,
flush toilets

PARKING: At campsites only

FEE: $14 per night (varies
by season)

ELEVATION: 777 feet

RESTRICTIONS: Pets: Must be
attended and on
leash shorter than 6
feet; clean up after
pet
Fires: Use camp-
stoves and fire-
places; deadwood
within 100 yards of
campground may be
used
Alcohol: Permitted
Vehicles: Up to 30
feet
Other: Tent pads
required; quiet time
10 p.m.–6 a.m.;
campsite capacity is
6 people, 2 vehicles;
firearms prohibited.

rant parking lot to the James River Visitor Center, located just south of the campground along the James River. It crosses the creek twice before intersecting with the 0.9-mile Otter Lake Trail, which in turn loops around this small body of water.

The Otter Creek Campground works well as a base camp from which to explore the area or as a stopover on your way north or south. Plan to pack your bicycle, if for no other reason than just to ride the paved road that follows the undulations of the famed Blue Ridge Mountains. Paddling on the James, hiking on the Appalachian Trail that crosses US 501 just south of the campground, and mountain biking in the surrounding George Washington and Jefferson National Forests are all within a 15-minute drive. The Appalachian Trail and six others crisscross the 11,500-acre James River Face and adjoining Thunder Ridge Wilderness Areas just south of the James River. Nineteen miles of trails await mountain bikers at the South Pedlar ATV trail system, located a short distance west of the campground on US 501. Cyclists note that bikes may not be ridden on trails alongside the Blue Ridge Parkway, only on paved areas.

The James River follows the course of Virginia history, just as it has served as a major west-to-east transportation conduit since the first settlers followed it from the Chesapeake Bay to the site of Jamestown in 1607. The original plan was for the river to extend from Richmond to the Ohio River, but the James and Kanawha Canal only made it as far west as Buchanan, Virginia. Plan to cross the walkway over the James River and visit the rebuilt Lock No. 7 opposite the Otter Creek Visitor Center. The Battery Creek lock is typical of the 90 locks that were constructed on the canal. This one in particular operated from 1851–1880, but the first section of the canal system was built at the falls in

PEAKS OF OTTER
CAMPGROUND

Peaks of Otter offers a tremendous place to camp for those touring the Blue Ridge Parkway.

THE **MOUNTAINS OF THE BLUE RIDGE,** and of these the Peaks of Otter, are thought to be of a greater height, measured from their base, than any others in our country, and perhaps in North America," so said Thomas Jefferson in his only book, *Notes on the State of Virginia*. Given his expertise in architecture, law, politics, languages, and other fields, we'll have to forgive this bit of overstatement regarding the relative heights of Sharp Top and Flat Top, which stand at 3,875 feet and 4,001 feet, respectively. Given the manner in which they stand apart so geographically from their surroundings, it's easy to see how Charlottesville's favorite son could have embellished their stature a bit.

However, it's difficult to overstate the beauty of the 469-mile Blue Ridge Parkway that stretches from Afton Mountain in Virginia to Cherokee, North Carolina. It's surely one of the most beautiful roads in America; and the Peaks of Otter Campground, located at milepost 86, offers a tremendous place to pitch a tent for those passing through or intent on this as their final destination. Across the road is the picturesque Peaks of Otter Lodge, its reflection mirrored by Abbott Lake. You may want to sample the renowned bounty at the lodge should you tire of camp fare.

The campground's 144 sites are divided among three loops designated as A, B, and the trailer loop. If you've gotten fed up with campgrounds that offer larger, more private, or more abundant sites for RV users, then you'll love the campground at the Peaks of Otter. There are only 52 sites in the trailer loop, with an additional 4 trailer sites in Loop A. The

RATINGS

Beauty: ✿ ✿ ✿
Site privacy: ✿ ✿ ✿
Spaciousness: ✿ ✿ ✿ ✿
Quiet: ✿ ✿ ✿ ✿
Security: ✿ ✿ ✿
Cleanliness: ✿ ✿ ✿ ✿

MAP

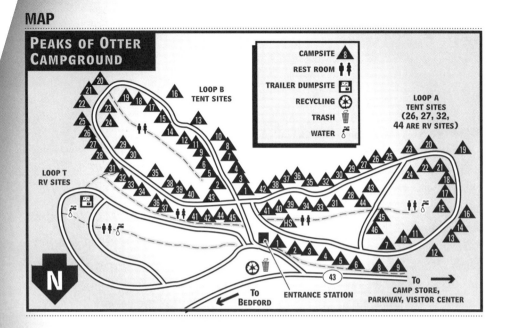

PEAKS OF OTTER CAMPGROUND

Legend:
- CAMPSITE 8
- REST ROOM
- TRAILER DUMPSITE
- RECYCLING
- TRASH
- WATER

LOOP B TENT SITES

LOOP A TENT SITES (26, 27, 32, 44 ARE RV SITES)

LOOP T RV SITES

N

To BEDFORD

ENTRANCE STATION

To CAMP STORE, PARKWAY, VISITOR CENTER

GETTING THERE

Take the Blue Ridge Parkway to its intersection with VA 43 at milepost 86, and go 0.25 mile south on VA 43 to the campground entrance.

the top. You can also pick up several trails at the visitor center, located on the other side of the Blue Ridge Parkway from the campground. These include the 0.8-mile Elk Run Trail, the 2.1-mile Johnson Farm Trail, and the 3.3-mile Harkening Hill Trail, all of which are loops. A number of other trails adjoin the Appalachian Trail and are accessible some 5 miles south of the peaks on the Blue Ridge Parkway.

KEY INFORMATION

ADDRESS: Lake Robertson Campground
106 Lake Robertson Drive
Lexington, VA 24450

OPERATED BY: Rockbridge County Parks and Recreation

INFORMATION: (540) 463-4164

WEB SITE: www.co.rockbridge.va.us/departments/lake_robertson.htm

OPEN: April 1–end of November

SITES: 53

EACH SITE HAS: Picnic table, electric and water hookups, and fire ring

ASSIGNMENT: By reservation or on arrival

REGISTRATION: By reservation or on arrival

FACILITIES: Water, hot showers, flush toilets, camp store, pay phone, laundry, and drink machines

PARKING: At campsites, max 2 vehicles

FEE: $20 per night for tent campers; $24 per night for trailers

ELEVATION: 1,540 feet

RESTRICTIONS: Pets: Must be on leash, attended, and quiet at all times; pet-walking area, must clean up after pet.
Fires: Confine to campstoves and fire rings
Alcohol: Prohibited
Vehicles: No limit
Other: Site capacity 6 people, 2 tents. No gas motors allowed.

The campground is located behind the camp store and across the park's main drive from the lake. Situated in a grove of trees along a single loop, there is little privacy between sites but ample shade from spring through summer. The campground slopes gently uphill with plenty of space between sites, especially those around the volleyball court at the top of the hill. Sites 26 through 30 surround the grassy hilltop and are a little farther from the park's other activities, while sites 20, 21, 23, and 25 are nearby along the edge of the campground road. The outer loop is sometimes closed in late October and November due to freezing. Tent campers should be sure to bring a ground cloth and mattress pad because several of the tent pads are gravel.

Those familiar with Virginia politics may recognize the name of deceased U.S. Senator A. Willis Robertson, for whom this park is named. He was a Lexington resident and co-sponsored the Federal Aid in Wildlife Restoration Program, which has been credited with funneling billions of dollars to states for wildlife restoration work. Most of us are better acquainted with the senator's prominent son, evangelist and politician Pat Robertson. This area is, as mentioned, ripe with history and natural beauty.

Surrounding Rockbridge County is named for Natural Bridge, a spectacular 215-foot high arch eroded out of limestone by Cedar Creek. Plan to take a picnic lunch to nearby Goshen Pass, an awesome gorge where the Maury River has carved a path over time through the Allegheny Mountains. Lexington is the home of Washington and Lee University and the Virginia Military Institute. Stonewall Jackson owned a home here, and Civil War skirmishes were fought in the surrounding area.

You could use Lake Robertson campground as a base from which to explore the rich history and beauty of Rockbridge County and Lexington, located just 10 miles away. You could, however, just

MORRIS HILL CAMPGROUND

> *The northern end of Lake Moomaw is bordered by the 13,428-acre Gathright Wildlife Management Area.*

ON A HILLTOP NEAR the southern end of manmade Lake Moomaw, Morris Hill Campground features a loop of 39 unreserved tent sites around a heavily wooded ravine. A nearby spur has 16 reservable sites that can house tents or RVs. Three of the reservable sites are categorized as wheelchair-accessible and are located next to one of the three bathhouses.

All of the sites are situated in an area of mature hardwoods with enough low-growth vegetation to provide privacy between campsites. There is also ample space between campsites so that you won't feel that you're camping cheek to jowl. The central ravine adds significantly to the feeling of being nestled in the nearby George Washington National Forest.

A short walk via the Morris Mill Trail (0.75-mile point-to-point) or the Fortney Branch Trail (1.3-mile point-to-point) will take you to the lake. This 2,500-acre lake straddles the Alleghany–Bath County line, and recreational facilities are managed by two National Forest ranger districts. The southern end, where Morris Hill Campground is located, is managed by the James River District; the northern end is managed by the Warm Springs District.

Lake Moomaw was formed in 1981 by the construction of the Gathright Dam. The dam's cooling tower keeps the Jackson River and Lake Moomaw waters temperate even in late summer, giving the region some of the best trout fishing in Virginia. The area also supports abundant wildlife including wild turkeys, white-tailed deer, and the occasional black bear. The average depth of the lake is 80 feet,

RATINGS

Beauty: ☆ ☆ ☆
Site privacy: ☆ ☆ ☆ ☆
Spaciousness: ☆ ☆ ☆ ☆
Quiet: ☆ ☆ ☆
Security: ☆ ☆ ☆
Cleanliness: ☆ ☆ ☆

MAP

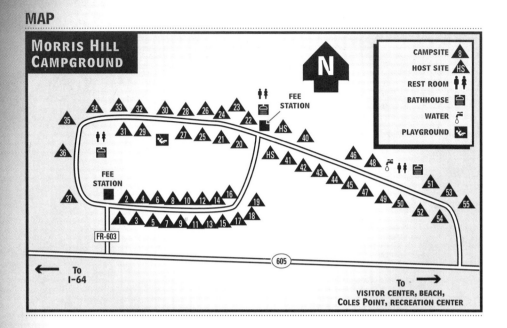

GETTING THERE

From I-64, take Exit 16 and follow US 220 north for 4 miles. Turn left onto SR 687 and follow it for 3 miles. Turn left onto SR 641 and go 1 mile before turning right onto SR 666. Continue for 5 miles and then turn right onto SR 605. You'll find FDR 603, the entrance to the Morris Hill Campground, 2 miles ahead.

I'd be remiss if I didn't mention these camping options so close by, but given the choice, I'd much prefer to pitch my tent in the serene seclusion of Morris Hill.

springs often lead to the development of caves, so it's no surprise that the abundance of springs in rural Bath County is part of the state's longest cave network, the Butler–Sinking Creek system. Bob Gulden, a dedicated spelunker and cave mapmaker from Maryland, has listed some 17 miles of passages for this system.

Even if you don't try the healing waters, there's little doubt that a weekend spent camping nearby has got to leave you better off than when you arrived. A well-worn but unmarked trail leads from behind the campground's SST (sweet-smellin' toilet) to the mossy groundwater surface from which Bubbling Spring emanates, providing the source for Lick Run along the edge of the campground. This narrow creek provides a perfect touch to the woodland setting, as well as a convenient spot to fish for trout. Pads Creek is another local stream that offers some challenges for those who like their streams narrow and their catch wary.

In addition to trout fishing, there are plenty of opportunities for other outdoor pursuits in this section of the George Washington and Jefferson National Forests. Hikers can enjoy the nearby 3-mile (one way) strenuous hike of Rough Mountain in the 9,300-acre Rough Mountain Wilderness. Numerous trails start just west of the Cowpasture River and north of Douthat State Park. You can relish the quiet at Bubbling Springs and still hike or bike the extensive trail system at Douthat. The charming country towns of Millboro Springs and Goshen are both worth a visit, and Goshen Pass, a 3-mile stretch of VA 39, offers a breathtaking alternate route back to the Shenandoah Valley.

The southeastern end of the 33,697-acre Goshen–Little North Mountain Wildlife Management Area is located just east of the Bubbling Springs Campground. Wildlife management areas are maintained by the Virginia Department of

DOUTHAT
STATE PARK

This CCC-constructed lakeside getaway in far western Virginia lies in a valley between Beards and Middle Mountains.

SCENIC **DOUTHAT STATE PARK** was deemed one of the nation's top ten state parks by the *Outside Family Vacation Guide* in 1999 and in that same year was honored with a Centennial Medallion from the American Society of Landscape Architects. These 4,493 acres were part of a land grant given to Robert Douthat by Governor Robert Brooke in 1795. In 1936, Douthat became one of the original six parks to comprise the Virginia State Park system. This CCC-constructed lakeside getaway lies in a valley between Beards and Middle Mountains, through which Wilson Creek and SR 629 run. The neighboring peaks reach heights of 3,000 feet while the lake is nestled at 1,146 feet.

The park's Depression-era beginnings led to its designation as a Registered National Historic Landmark. Great fishing in the 50-acre lake, rental cabins, and more than 40 miles of hiking trails across the adjacent mountainsides are but a few of the attractions that draw large numbers of vacationers out to this rustic setting. Stone walls, log pavilions, and wrought-iron attachments all speak to the CCC craftsmanship. Another popular stop is the recently renovated Lakeview Restaurant and Country Store.

Douthat's 74 campsites are divided among three campgrounds: Lakeside, Beaver Dam, and White Oak. Tent campers usually head for nonelectric Lakeside Campground, which is closest to the lake. The sites have no wooded privacy barriers, but the views of the lake and neighboring mountains are worth the compromise. Lakeside Campground is located between Beaver Dam Campground to the north and White Oak Campground to the south. Its

RATINGS

Beauty: ✿ ✿ ✿ ✿
Site privacy: ✿ ✿ ✿
Spaciousness: ✿ ✿ ✿
Quiet: ✿ ✿ ✿
Security: ✿ ✿ ✿
Cleanliness: ✿ ✿ ✿ ✿

MAP

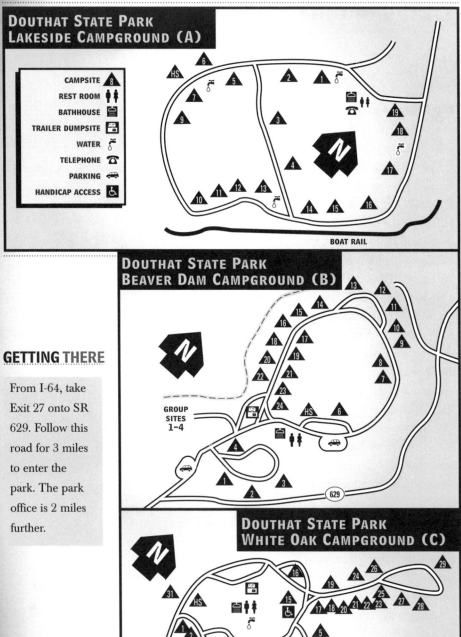

GETTING THERE

From I-64, take Exit 27 onto SR 629. Follow this road for 3 miles to enter the park. The park office is 2 miles further.

KEY INFORMATION

ADDRESS: Hidden Valley
Campground
Warm Springs
Ranger District
US 220 South
Route 2, Box 30
Hot Springs, VA
24445

OPERATED BY: U.S. Forest Service

INFORMATION: (540) 839-2521

WEB SiTE: www.southern
region.fs.fed.us/gwj

OPEN: Mid-March–end of
November

SITES: 30

EACH SITE HAS: Picnic table, fire
grill, and lantern
pole

ASSIGNMENT: First come, first
served; no reser-
vations

REGISTRATION: Self-registration on
site

FACILITIES: Water and vault
toilet

PARKING: At campsite

FEE: $6 per night

ELEVATION: 1,800 feet

RESTRICTIONS: Pets: On leash only
and not allowed in
swimming areas
Fires: In fire rings,
stoves, or grills only
Alcohol: May be
consumed responsi-
bly at campsite
Vehicles: 25-foot
limit
Other: Do not carve,
chop, or damage any
live trees; keep
noise at a reasonable
level; length of stay
no more than 14
days in 30-day
period; quiet time
10 p.m.–7 a.m.

deer season. Although Virginia's Department of Game and Inland Fisheries went to a year-round trout season several years back, there's still a contingent of anglers who make their way to this stretch of the Jackson River in early spring out of habit. Almost any other time of year, however, you're likely to arrive at Hidden Valley Campground to your choice of campsites and few neighbors. The campground's 30 sites are shaded and set along a single loop. Vegetation between the large campsites provides a considerable amount of privacy.

The Jackson River is an excellent trout stream and is accessible via the Hidden Valley Trail, which starts at the campground and follows the river for 6.2 miles—including several stream crossings sans bridges. This trail is also the start of a popular 12-mile mountain bike loop that circles back on FDR 241-2 past the mansion. Other trails include the 0.6-mile Lower Lost Woman Trail and the 1-mile Upper Lost Woman Trail, both accessible from the campground.

The Warm Springs Ranger District is a beautiful part of Virginia, and although you can have a dandy time exploring Hidden Valley without getting back into your car, plan to explore the Warm Springs/Hot Springs area. No visit would be complete without a healthy dip into Warm Springs, located at the intersections of VA 220 and VA 39. There are separate facilities for men and women, with the women's structure dating to 1836 and the men's to 1761, making it one of the oldest spas in the country. Indigenous people are thought to have frequented these springs as far back as 9,000 years ago.

Western Virginia was once famous for its healing springs, and wealthy urbanites spent their summers allowing the waters to cure what ailed them—as well as to escape mosquito-borne diseases and socialize at the resorts. Hot Springs was initially developed by early settlers Thomas Bullet and brothers Thomas and Andrew Lewis in 1766. This

CAVE MOUNTAIN LAKE CAMPGROUND

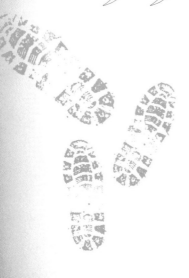

This area of the Shenandoah Valley is rife with limestone deposits, sinkholes, and the accompanying caves.

SPLENDIDLY NESTLED at the foot of the peaks of the Blue Ridge Mountains is Cave Mountain Lake Recreation Area. The campground is a short walk through the woods away from the lake, which means that you won't get a view of the water from your tent flap. Fortunately, this separation gives campers some privacy from visitors who come for the day to swim in the seven-acre lake and feed at the adjoining picnic area.

The entrance road climbs and winds through a forest of pine, hemlock, and assorted hardwoods, before dropping down into the wooded camping area. The sites are spread out along a large loop and small spur with sites 36, 37, and 38 designated as walk-in sites that offer a higher degree of privacy than the rest. All of the sites, however, are spacious and the tall foliage creates privacy for each site. Tent pads consist of a fine gravel surface. The camping area features flush toilets and water hydrants, and showers are nearby at the beach rest room. Back Run courses its way through the campground before entering the Cave Mountain Lake. Back Run is usually placid and delightful but can overflow its banks after heavy rains. Plan accordingly.

Located a short distance from Natural Bridge Caverns and Natural Bridge itself, this area of the Shenandoah Valley is rife with limestone deposits, sinkholes, and the accompanying caves. The 90-foot Natural Bridge is an imposing limestone arch that stands 215 feet above the gorge carved out by Cedar Creek. Some consider it to be one of the seven natural wonders of the world. Certainly it is one of the wonders of the Shenandoah Valley. First discovered

RATINGS

Beauty: ✿ ✿ ✿
Site privacy: ✿ ✿ ✿ ✿
Spaciousness: ✿ ✿ ✿ ✿
Quiet: ✿ ✿ ✿
Security: ✿ ✿ ✿ ✿
Cleanliness: ✿ ✿ ✿ ✿ ✿

MAP

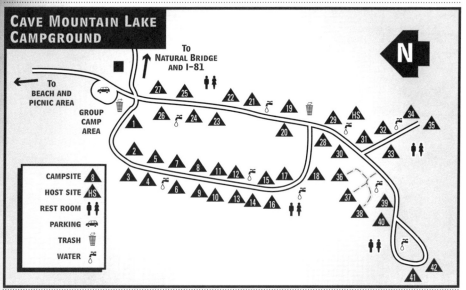

CAVE MOUNTAIN LAKE CAMPGROUND

To NATURAL BRIDGE AND I-81

To BEACH AND PICNIC AREA

GROUP CAMP AREA

CAMPSITE	8
HOST SITE	HS
REST ROOM	👫
PARKING	🚐
TRASH	🗑
WATER	🚰

GETTING THERE

From I-81, take Exit 180 to US 11 to Natural Bridge. Follow VA 130 East from Natural Bridge for 3 miles then turn right onto SR 759. Follow SR 759 for 3.2 miles and turn right onto SR 781. Continue for another 1.6 miles to the entrance for Cave Mountain Lake Recreation Area.

its natural beauty and relative seclusion make it a worthwhile destination for those looking for solace.

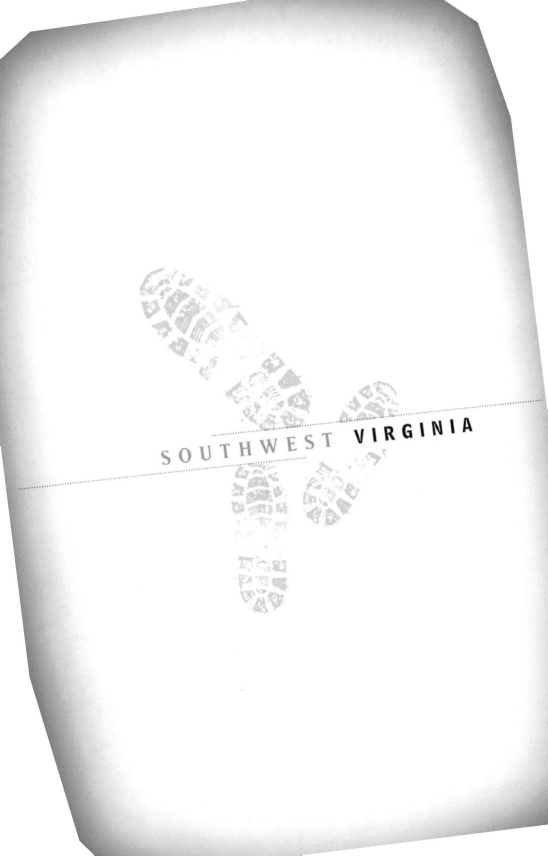

SOUTHWEST VIRGINIA

ADDRESS: Claytor Lake State Park
4400 State Park Road
Dublin, VA 24084

OPERATED BY: Virginia Department of Conservation and Recreation

INFORMATION: (540) 643-2500

WEB SITE: www.dcr.state.va.us/parks

OPEN: April 1–December 1

SITES: 110

EACH SITE HAS: Picnic table, fire grill, and lantern pole

ASSIGNMENT: First come, first served

REGISTRATION: (800) 933-PARK or on arrival

FACILITIES: Flush toilets and hot showers; pay phone and drink machines at marina

PARKING: 2 vehicles in addition to camping unit; extra parking available

FEE: $18 per night; $23 with electricity and water

ELEVATION: 1,900 feet

RESTRICTIONS: Pets: Must be on short leash or enclosed
Fires: Contained to camp stoves and fire rings
Alcohol: Public use or display is prohibited
Vehicles: Up to 35 feet
Other: Swimming only in designated areas; no cutting of trees; no washing dishes in rest room sinks

minimal understory for privacy between sites. In this respect, have a look at sites A9–A27, which are flat but laid out on a hillside.

Loop D has a different feel to A, B, or C. In addition to being positioned along a flat open area, it's the only one without delineated tent pads. So you have the option to pitch your tent on terra firma, either in the open or among groves of pine trees. Loop D sites are laid out along three lines, but D30–D34 are the most secluded, with the dirt access road in front and a buffer of pine trees behind them. Despite its appearance as more conducive to tent camping than the other loops, it's also the only one with electrical hookups and is geared towards RVs. Go figure.

The park has five picnic shelters and one gazebo that are available for rent, and 3 miles of trails for easy walks through the woods. You can pick up the 1.6-mile Claytor Lake Trail across from site C4, while the 0.6-mile Shady Ridge Trail is accessible from the picnic area. Mountain bikers may want to use Claytor Lake State Park to ride on the 57-mile New River Trail, part of which runs along Claytor Lake.

Be sure to stop by the historic Howe House, built between 1876 and 1879 by Haven B. Howe. Besides being a Civil War veteran, Virginia legislator, and talented woodworker, Howe was an early environmentalist who worked to end pollution of the New River by iron ore smelting plants. He was also a proponent of conservation-oriented farming. Howe House was built with brick that had been kiln-dried on the property along with timber felled from the surrounding woods. It now houses the park's visitor center and administrative offices. It contains hands-on exhibits that focus on lake ecology and fish life as well as the park's Discovery Center, which offers summer environmental education programs.

GRAYSON HIGHLANDS STATE PARK

> *The overall feeling is that you're clinging to the roof of the Old Dominion.*

WITH ELEVATIONS UP TO 5,089 feet, Grayson Highlands is the loftiest state park in Virginia. From the highest point at the Pinnacles you'll find breathtaking views of surrounding mountains, including Mount Rogers (5,729 feet), the tallest peak in Virginia. The overall feeling is not that you're on an isolated elevation but more like you're clinging to the roof of the Old Dominion. Originally known as Mount Rogers State Park, Grayson Highlands became part of the state system in 1965. As you enter the park from US 58 at 3,698 feet and ascend to the visitor center at 4,953 feet, you get the feeling that you're climbing into heaven. And for many campers, that's exactly where you're headed.

The park office is on the left after the contact station. The campground turnoff is another 2.5 miles by the overnight parking area for backpackers. Grayson Highlands has the distinction of being one of two Virginia State Parks through which the 2,172-mile Appalachian Trail passes on its way between Maine and Georgia. It's a popular spot with thru-hikers as well as for those looking to accumulate some AT mileage.

The campground is isolated, its sites clustered around a grassy bald knoll. The 73 sites are positioned along two interlocking loops, with considerable differences in privacy and exposure. Past the first bathhouse, the woods become more invasive. On top of elevations such as this, however, trees have a tough time getting much height. Given a choice, it's definitely worth a drive around to pick out a good site, especially if spending a few days

RATINGS

Beauty: ✿ ✿ ✿ ✿
Site privacy: ✿ ✿ ✿
Spaciousness: ✿ ✿ ✿
Quiet: ✿ ✿ ✿
Security: ✿ ✿ ✿
Cleanliness: ✿ ✿ ✿ ✿

MAP

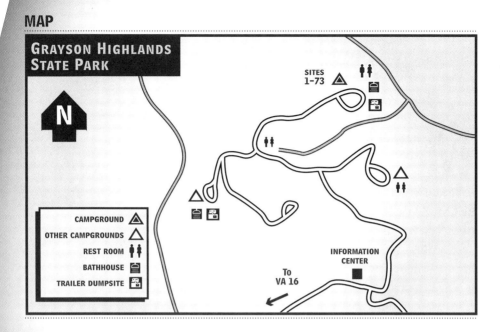

GRAYSON HIGHLANDS STATE PARK

N

SITES 1-73

To VA 16

INFORMATION CENTER

CAMPGROUND

OTHER CAMPGROUNDS

REST ROOM

BATHHOUSE

TRAILER DUMPSITE

GETTING THERE

From I-81, take Exit 45 at Marion and drive 33 miles south on VA 16. Turn right onto US 58 in the community of Volney and continue 8 miles to the park's entrance.

views from this lofty point. Mount Rogers is capped by spruce trees and offers no views at all.

Many festivals take place at Grayson Highlands State Park from March through October. The park gets crowded so plan your trip accordingly. Also, keep in mind that the weather can change rapidly here, so pack for extremes of temperature. One balmy Easter Sunday I hiked around the park in shorts and a T-shirt only to be snowed on that evening.

ADDRESS: New River Trail State Park
176 Orphanage Drive
Foster Falls, VA 24360

OPERATED BY: Virginia Department of Conservation and Recreation

INFORMATION: (276) 699-6778

WEB SITE: www.dcr.state.va.us/parks

OPEN: Year-round

SITES: 12, plus 9 group sites that may be rented individually as overflow

EACH SITE HAS: Picnic table, fire ring, lantern post, bike rack

ASSIGNMENT: Assigned in advance

REGISTRATION: Reservations required (800) 933-PARK; same day reservations accepted

FACILITIES: Vault toilets, water (water turned off in winter)

PARKING: Park in lot, walk or bike to site

FEE: $13 per night

ELEVATION: 1,900 feet

RESTRICTIONS: Pets: Must be on short leash or enclosed; $3 per night
Fires: Confined to fire pits and camp stoves
Alcohol: Public use or display prohibited
Vehicles: None
Other: Maximum stay 14-days in a 30-day period, no more than 6 people per site.

oldest river in the world and flows north. The average width of the park is only 80 feet.

The 765-acre park runs through Grayson, Carroll, Wythe, and Pulaski counties. It features two tunnels, three major bridges, and nearly 30 smaller bridges and trestles. It can be used by cyclists, hikers, and horseback riders and features a link to the Virginia Creeper Trail. New River Trail links up to several other recreation areas, including Mount Rogers National Recreational Area, four Department of Game and Inland Fisheries boat launches, a town park in Fries, and the 150-year-old Shot Tower Historical State Park. Shot Tower is a 75-foot tall structure in which lead was melted and poured down a sieve into a kettle of water, to make ammunition for early settlers. Additionally, Claytor Lake State Park and Grayson Highlands State Park are just minutes away.

New River Trail is home to several events and festivals throughout the year. Most notable is the New River Trail Challenge, a late September triathlon in which participants bike 40 miles to Foster Falls. From there, they take canoes and paddle 12 miles to Allisonia, where they finish the race with a 13.1-mile half-marathon run. The canoe portion of the race includes Class I and II rapids.

Cliffview Campground is also in New River Trail State Park, and is located near Galax, 20 miles from Millrace Campground. Vehicles must be parked a mile from the campground and campers must hike, bike, or horseback ride in from the ranger station. There are ten campsites for hikers and bikers, along with three sites that feature hitching posts and are designated horseback sites. Horseback riders may park horse trailers at the Cliffview, Draper, Fries, Pulaski, or Foster Falls park entrances. Cliffview campers should reserve ahead and proceed directly to their sites, while Millrace campers can register at the Foster Falls

HUNGRY MOTHER
STATE PARK

> *Swimming, boating, and fishing for northern pike are just a few of the possibilities here.*

HUNGRY MOTHER STATE PARK is one of the original six parks that formed the nucleus of Virginia's state system in 1936. The legend behind this park's name is as colorful as the foliage that wraps around this setting in the fall. Back in Virginia's past when relations between settlers and Native Americans were at an ebb, it is said that a party of Native American warriors destroyed several settlements south of what is now the park on the New River. Molly Marley and her child escaped the attacks but were taken captive. They were eventually able to escape, subsisting on wild berries as they made their way through the wilderness. Molly finally collapsed while her child continued by following a creek. When the child found help, its only words were, "hungry, mother." The search party followed the creek and found Molly dead at the base of a mountain. The mountain became Molly's Knob and the creek was named Hungry Mother Creek. The creek was dammed in 1930 to form Hungry Mother Lake.

The park is located 4 miles from Marion on Virginia 16, which passes through the park boundaries. It contains 43 sites distributed over three campgrounds. Campground A is located alongside VA 16. This campground sits on a small field with no vegetation between sites and offers little in the way of atmosphere, privacy, or seclusion. Campground B is located across VA 348 and is RV-oriented. Its 21 sites have electric and water hookups and are situated close to each other along a maze of hard surface roads.

RATINGS

Beauty: ✿ ✿ ✿ ✿
Site privacy: ✿ ✿ ✿ ✿
Spaciousness: ✿ ✿ ✿ ✿
Quiet: ✿ ✿ ✿ ✿
Security: ✿ ✿ ✿
Cleanliness: ✿ ✿ ✿ ✿

MAP

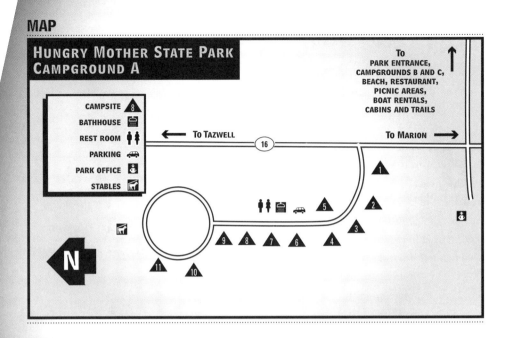

HUNGRY MOTHER STATE PARK CAMPGROUND A

To PARK ENTRANCE, CAMPGROUNDS B AND C, BEACH, RESTAURANT, PICNIC AREAS, BOAT RENTALS, CABINS AND TRAILS

CAMPSITE
BATHHOUSE
REST ROOM
PARKING
PARK OFFICE
STABLES

To Tazwell
16
To Marion

N

GETTING THERE

From I-81, take Exit 47 heading toward Marion on US 11. Turn right in Marion onto VA 16 and continue for 4 miles to the park's entrance.

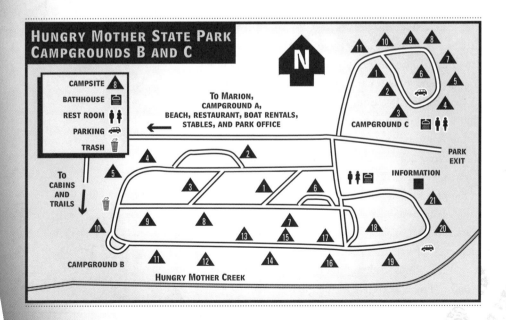

HUNGRY MOTHER STATE PARK CAMPGROUNDS B AND C

N

CAMPSITE
BATHHOUSE
REST ROOM
PARKING
TRASH

To MARION, CAMPGROUND A, BEACH, RESTAURANT, BOAT RENTALS, STABLES, AND PARK OFFICE

CAMPGROUND C

PARK EXIT

INFORMATION

To CABINS AND TRAILS

CAMPGROUND B

HUNGRY MOTHER CREEK

ADDRESS: Breaks Interstate
Park
P.O. Box 100
Breaks, VA 24607

OPERATED BY: Breaks Interstate
Commission

INFORMATION: (276) 865-4413

WEB SITE: www.breakspark.
com

OPEN: April 1–October 31

SITES: 122

EACH SITE HAS: Picnic table and fire
grill

ASSIGNMENT: First come, first
served

REGISTRATION: On arrival, no reservations

FACILITIES: Camp store, laundry,
vending machines,
restaurant, flush toi-
lets, showers

PARKING: 2 vehicles in addition to camping unit
at site

FEE: $9 per night; $15
with electricity and
water

ELEVATION: 1,600 feet

RESTRICTIONS: Pets: Must be on
leash
Fires: Build only in
designated areas
Alcohol: Prohibited
Vehicles: Up to 40
feet
Other: Maximum 6
people per site

gorge is covered in so much forest that the drama of the scene is tempered. It appears to be a panoramic wooded valley rather than a canyon chiseled out by erosion. Regardless, it offers stunning views along with a variety of outdoor adventures.

Seventeen miles of trails offer 13 miles of hiking. Most of the trails are short, but can be combined to form longer treks. The longest is the 3-mile Mountain Bike Trail, but bicycles are not allowed on any of the other trails. The park convenience store rents bikes, which can also be used on park roads. Grassy Overlook Trail can be accessed from between sites 10 and 11 in Section B of the campground. Overlook Trail, which hugs the edge of cliffs, is popular in spring and fall. Other activities include horseback riding and pool swimming, along with boating and fishing on the central 12-acre Laurel Lake or on the trout-stocked Russell Fork River. Additionally, whitewater rafting is popular in October when water released from Flanagan Reservoir creates Class IV to Class VI rapids.

Also popular, especially with non-hikers, is the nearby Cumberland Mountain View Drive. It is a 19-mile panoramic trip along SR 611, between Breaks Interstate Park and Clintwood, Virginia. Parts of the road are unpaved, and there are several sharp turns, so allow several hours for the trip.

Daniel Boone is credited with discovering Breaks. He is mentioned in the small museum located at the visitor center. Exhibits also detail the unique geology that caused the sandstone erosion, as well as the formation of coal and process of coal mining—past and present—in the local hills. Just outside the visitor center is a working mill and a non-working moonshine still. The region is full of folklore about mountain folk, including the infamous Hatfield-McCoy feud, which is said to have occurred nearby.

CAVE SPRINGS
RECREATION AREA

> *The quarter-acre, spring-fed pond at Cave Springs is a great destination.*

FAR OUT IN THE SOUTHWEST corner of Virginia is an area known for coal production but largely overlooked by the rest of the state. Its topography of horizontal Appalachian Plateau sandstone identifies it less with Virginia and more with neighboring Kentucky, Tennessee, and West Virginia. Local residents are known for their tenacity in carving out lives from largely inhospitable landscapes. Early timber and mining efforts stripped many of these mountains, and the Forest Service bought land for the Clinch Ranger District to protect the headwaters of the Tennessee River. Visit this little-known region, and you'll be amazed by the natural beauty that lies in this obscure corner of the Old Dominion.

Cave Springs Recreation Area is one of those scarcely visited gems harbored in Virginia's National Forests. It lies at the foot of Stone Mountain, which is part of Cumberland Mountain, forming the border with Kentucky. Most people don't even know that Virginia shares a border with the Bluegrass State. While few Virginians make the drive out to the Clinch Ranger District, those lucky enough to live nearby or in the neighboring states of Kentucky and Tennessee can savor this outstanding camping destination.

After passing through a rolling agricultural landscape, you'll find this wooded oasis where dense stands of holly hug the quarter-acre spring-fed pond. Cave Springs is particularly appealing during the heat of the summer. The entire recreation area is shaded by a canopy of hemlocks, and the spring-fed pond stays below 72°F. Those

RATINGS

Beauty: ✿ ✿ ✿ ✿
Site privacy: ✿ ✿ ✿ ✿
Spaciousness: ✿ ✿ ✿ ✿ ✿
Quiet: ✿ ✿ ✿
Security: ✿ ✿ ✿
Cleanliness: ✿ ✿ ✿

MAP

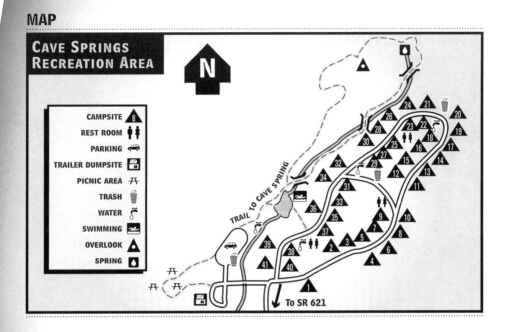

CAVE SPRINGS RECREATION AREA

N

CAMPSITE	8
REST ROOM	
PARKING	
TRAILER DUMPSITE	
PICNIC AREA	
TRASH	
WATER	
SWIMMING	
OVERLOOK	
SPRING	

TRAIL TO CAVE SPRING

To SR 621

GETTING THERE

From Big Stone Gap, follow US Alt. 58 west for 3 miles to SR 621. Turn right onto SR 621 and follow it for 6.5 miles to the sign for Cave Springs.

waters, hike the mountains, and discover all that's so refreshing about a part of Virginia that many Virginians have forgotten.

ADDRESS:	Hurricane Campground Mount Rogers National Recreation Area 3714 VA 16 Marion, VA 24354
OPERATED BY:	U.S. Forest Service
INFORMATION:	(276) 783-5196
WEB SITE:	www.southern region.fs.fed.us/gwj/mr/campgrounds
OPEN:	April–October
SITES:	24 single, 6 double
EACH SITE HAS:	Picnic table, fire grill, lantern pole
ASSIGNMENT:	First come, first served
REGISTRATION:	On site
FACILITIES:	Flush toilets, warm showers
PARKING:	At campsite
FEE:	$14 per night single; $26 per night double
ELEVATION:	2,880 feet
RESTRICTIONS:	Pets: Must be on leash and attended Fires: Use available grills Alcohol: Prohibited Vehicles: Up to 22 feet Other: Length of stay no more than 14 days in a 30-day period; no cutting live trees; quiet time 10 p.m.–6 a.m.

benefit of limited drive-by traffic.

Mount Rogers National Recreation Area is geared towards recreation. In addition to its seclusion, Hurricane Campground provides an excellent base camp from which to explore some outstanding trails and forest roads by foot, horse, or mountain bike.

The trailhead for the 1-mile Hurricane Knob Loop Trail is located at the entrance to the campground across from the information kiosk. The 9.6-mile Four Trails Circuit covers bits of the Dickey Knob, Comers Creek Falls, Iron Mountain, and Appalachian Trails as it winds its way through some of the Mount Rogers NRA's finest woodland scenery. For that matter, you can pick up a National Forest map and plan to walk for a given distance on either the Iron Mountain or Appalachian Trail, both of which are ubiquitous in this 115,000-acre recreation area. Sixty miles of AT carve their way through the Mount Rogers area.

Mountain bikes are not allowed on the Appalachian Trail; otherwise possibilities for two-wheel fun seem limitless. Back when the sport was still new to Virginia and other park agencies were not aware of its existence, the folks in this district of the Jefferson National Forest were bold enough to proclaim that "whoever invented mountain bicycles surely had the Mount Rogers National Recreation Area in mind!" Those looking for minimal challenge and maximum fun will head for the 33-mile (one-way) Virginia Creeper Trail, a converted railroad bed that runs (downhill) from Whitetop Mountain to the town of Damascus. The Iron Mountain Trail gets a lot of use from local mountain bikers as well as visitors looking for additional technical and aerobic challenges. Combine sections of the Iron Mountain Trail with gravel Forest Service roads to create your own loop, or pick up one of the several guides that detail tried and true loop rides. Sections

COMERS ROCK CAMPGROUND

> *Comers Rock is a suitable alternative for those seeking to be "far from the madding crowd."*

WITH SO MANY CAMPGROUNDS in the Mount Rogers National Recreation Area from which to choose, some might wonder why the low-budget Comers Rock Campground is included here. Its ten sites, vault toilet, and location away from the epicenter of outdoor activities in this 115,000-acre National Forest recreation area will probably not draw many campers from the larger and spiffier campgrounds, such as Beartree and Grindstone. But these qualities, in fact, make it a suitable camping alternative for those seeking to be "far from the madding crowds."

Located a short distance from US 21 on the eastern end of the Mount Rogers NRA, this campground sits along gravel FDR 57. The views from this road running along the ridgeline of Iron Mountain are nothing short of spectacular. Iron Mountain forms a recreational as well as a geologic spine for the area with this campground situated in a saddle with northern views across the adjacent 2,858-acre Little Dry Run Wilderness. The campsites are haphazardly arranged along a single loop with little vegetation between them, and some sites are not clearly marked. But they are all separated from each other with varied elevations that provide a modicum of privacy.

A trail next to the single vault toilet connects with the Virginia Highlands Horse Trail which meanders throughout Mount Rogers NRA along Iron Mountain. This section of the trail is designated multi-use, so hikers and mountain bikers can use the orange-blazed path to take off from their campsites for some outdoor exploration. Given that

RATINGS

Beauty: ✿ ✿ ✿
Site privacy: ✿ ✿
Spaciousness: ✿ ✿ ✿
Quiet: ✿ ✿ ✿
Security: ✿ ✿
Cleanliness: ✿ ✿ ✿

MAP

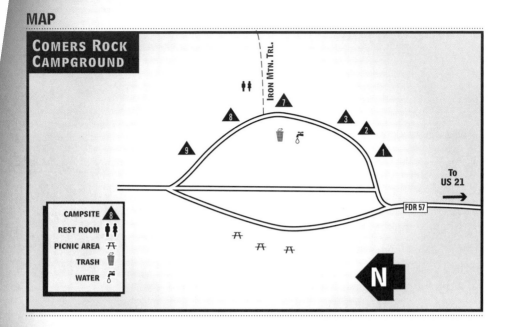

COMERS ROCK CAMPGROUND

IRON MTN. TRL.

To US 21 →

FDR 57

CAMPSITE	8
REST ROOM	👫
PICNIC AREA	⛩
TRASH	🗑
WATER	🚰

N

GETTING THERE

From Wytheville, take US 21 through Speedwell and turn right onto FDR 57 at the top of Iron Mountain. Go 4 miles to the campground.

Old Dominion, including 60 miles of Appalachian Trail. The AT goes right through the town of Damascus. Whatever your outdoor interests, you're sure to find places to enjoy it at Mount Rogers.

ADDRESS: Raven Cliff
Campground
Mount Rogers
National
Recreation Area
3714 VA 16
Marion, VA 24354

OPERATED BY: U.S. Forest Service

INFORMATION: (276) 783-5196

WEB SITE: www.southern
region.fs.fed.us/gwj/
mr/campgrounds

OPEN: Year-round

SITES: 20

EACH SITE HAS: Picnic table, fire
grill, lantern pole

ASSIGNMENT: First come, first
served

REGISTRATION: On site

FACILITIES: Vault toilet and
water

PARKING: At campsite and day-
use area

FEE: $5 per night

ELEVATION: 2,240 feet

RESTRICTIONS: Pets: Must be on
leash and attended
Fires: Use camp
stove or fire rings
Alcohol: Prohibited
Vehicles: Up to 32
feet
Other: Length of
stay no more than 14
days in a 30-day
period; Forest Ser-
vice does not plow
snow; no cutting live
trees; quiet time
10 p.m.–6 a.m.

the Iron Mountain Trail, Appalachian Trail, Virginia Creeper Trail, and others in the Mount Rogers Recreation Area—or you're just looking for a great, secluded campground in which to pitch your tent—then Raven Cliff could be the place for your next camping trip.

Take the 1-mile (out-and-back) walk along Cripple Creek on the Raven Cliff Furnace Trail to see the remains of the furnace, in use until the early 1900s. Iron ore was mixed with limestone and charcoal and combined under extreme temperatures to form "pigs," which were then shipped to Richmond and other sites for casting.

While Raven Cliff is far from the various trails and recreational attractions that the Mount Rogers NRA has to offer, mountain bikers enjoy a degree of comfort from Raven Cliff's relative proximity to the 57-mile New River State Park. Head south on VA 94, then turn left onto SR 602 to get onto the trail at the Byllesby Dam. The dam is near the southwestern prongs of the trail which end at Fries (pronounced "freeze") and Galax. Heading in a northeasterly direction on this converted railroad bed will also have you pedaling downhill for the better part of 30 miles toward the trail's northeastern terminus at Pulaski. The last 10 miles from Draper to Pulaski are on a slight uphill slope. In addition to largely avoiding vehicular traffic, one of the great advantages of rail-trail conversions such as the New River Trail is the modest gradient that you'll find. The downhills are enjoyable, and the uphills are very bearable.

Pedaling along this slight incline on the well-graded cinder surface is probably the easiest riding you're going to do. If you're planning an out-and-back, however, and a 60-miler sounds too ambitious, pedal from the Byllesby Dam at mile 37.3 to Shot Tower State Park at mile 25.2 along the New River Trail. This is a manageable 24-mile round

HIGH KNOB
RECREATION AREA

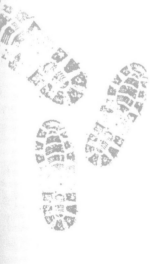

> *You'll want to make the 1.5-mile (one-way) assault on the observation tower at High Knob.*

WITH ITS SMALL SIZE, seclusion, absence of RV hookups, and small swimming hole located off by itself in the Clinch Ranger District of the George Washington and Jefferson Forest, remote High Knob Recreation Area is one of those amazing finds that you'll almost want to keep to yourself. But tell your friends—you wouldn't want to deprive them of the magnificent views from the lookout tower.

From the park entrance, it is a 1.7-mile drive down to the day-use section. This area can be lush with hemlocks, rhododendron, and an understory of ferns even when the rest of Virginia suffers from drought. Just before the driveway's end on the right side of the road is the trail leading to the High Knob Observation Tower. At the bottom of the driveway is the parking lot for the day-use area and lake on the left. The campground is located to the right, and features 13 single sites and one double site. Because of the narrow twisty roads leading up to and into the campground, you're not likely to be rubbing elbows with RVers, although RVs of up to 16 feet are welcome.

Located at an elevation of 3,800 feet, the 300-foot beach and four-acre "cold-water" spring-fed lake is guaranteed to provide a refreshing, if not shocking wake-up call, or a pleasant dip on a hot, summer afternoon. The ambient temperature in this region can be as much as 20 degrees cooler than the rest of Virginia, which campers appreciate during languid 100-degree-plus heat waves. The log and

RATINGS

Beauty: ✿ ✿ ✿ ✿
Site privacy: ✿ ✿ ✿ ✿
Spaciousness: ✿ ✿ ✿ ✿
Quiet: ✿ ✿ ✿ ✿ ✿
Security: ✿ ✿ ✿
Cleanliness: ✿ ✿ ✿ ✿ ✿

MAP

HIGH KNOB RECREATION AREA

To FDR 238

To HIGH KNOB TOWER

N

CAMPSITE	8
REST ROOM	🚹🚺
BATHHOUSE	🛁
PARKING	🚗
TRAILER DUMPSITE	
PICNIC AREA	🛆
AMPHITHEATER	📢

12 10 7
11 6
14 9 5
8 4
2
3 1

15

GROUP CAMPSITE

HS

DAY-USE AREA

HIGH KNOB LAKE

TRAIL AROUND HIGH KNOB LAKE

GETTING THERE

From Norton, go 3.7 miles south on SR 619. Turn left onto FDR 238 and follow it for 1.6 miles to the campground entrance.

gated Forest Service roads that lace the area. Before undertaking any exploration, be sure to pick up a copy of the Clinch Ranger District map from National Forest headquarters in Wise.

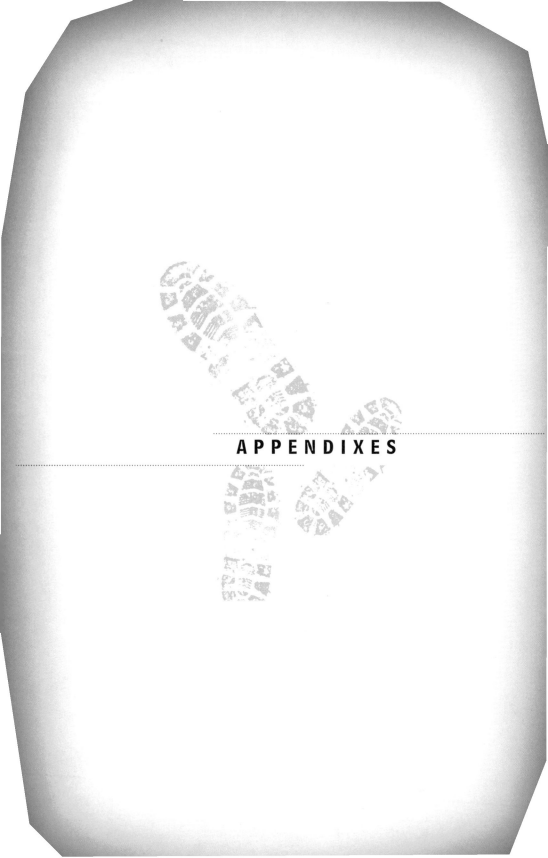

APPENDIXES

Except for the large and bulky items on this list, I keep a plastic storage container full of the essentials of car camping so that they're ready to go when I am. I make a last-minute check of the inventory, resupply anything that's low or missing, and away I go!

COOKING UTENSILS

Bottle opener

Bottles of salt, pepper, spices, sugar, cooking oil, and maple syrup in waterproof, spill-proof containers

Can opener

Corkscrew

Cups, plastic or tin

Dish soap (biodegradable), sponge, and towel

Flatware

Food of your choice

Frying pan

Fuel for stove

Matches in waterproof container

Plates

Pocketknife

Pot with lid

Spatula

Stove

Tin foil

Wooden spoon

FIRST AID KIT

Band-Aids

First aid cream

Gauze pads

Ibuprofen or aspirin

Insect repellent

Moleskin

Snakebite kit (if you're heading for desert conditions)

Sunscreen/lip balm

Tape, waterproof adhesive

SLEEPING GEAR

Pillow

Sleeping bag

Sleeping pad, inflatable or insuiated

Tent with ground tarp and rainfly

MISCELLANEOUS

Bath soap (biodegradable), washcloth, and towel

Camp chair

Candles

Cooler

Deck of cards

Fire starter

Flashlight with fresh batteries

Foul weather clothing

Paper towels

Plastic zip-top bags

Sunglasses

Toilet paper

Water bottle

Wool blanket

OPTIONAL

Barbecue grill

Binoculars

Books on bird, plant, and wildlife identification

Fishing rod and tackle

Hatchet

Lantern

Maps (road, topographic, trails, etc.)

The following is a partial list of agencies, associations, and organizations to write or call for information on outdoor recreation opportunities in Virginia.

BLUE RIDGE PARKWAY
199 Hemphill Knob Road
Asheville, NC 28803
(828) 298-0398
www.nps.gov/blri

GEORGE WASHINGTON AND JEFFERSON NATIONAL FORESTS
5162 Valleypointe Parkway
Roanoke, VA 24019
(540) 265-5100
www.southernregion.fs.fed.us/gwj

SHENANDOAH NATIONAL PARK
3655 US Highway East
Luray, VA 22835
(540) 999-3500
www.nps.gov/shen

VIRGINIA DEPARTMENT OF CONSERVATION AND RECREATION
203 Governor Street, Suite 213
Richmond, VA 23219
(800) 933-PARK
www.dcr.state.va.us

VIRGINIA DEPARTMENT OF GAME AND INLAND FISHERIES
4010 West Broad Street
Richmond, VA 23230
(804) 367-1000
www.dgif.state.va.us

APPENDIX C
SUGGESTED READING
AND REFERENCE

The Best of the Appalachian Trail Overnight Hikes. Logue, Victoria and Frank. Adkins, Leonard M., 2004.

The Best of the Appalachian Trail Day Hikes. Logue, Victoria and Frank. Adkins, Leonard M., 2004.

Civil War Virginia: Battleground for a Nation. Robertson, James I. University Press of Virginia, 1993.

Day and Overnight Hikes in the Shenandoah National Park. Molloy, Johnny. Menasha Ridge Press, 2003.

Highroad Guide to the Virginia Mountains. Winegar, Deane & Garvey. Longstreet Press, 2003.

Mountain Bike! Virginia. Porter, Randy Menasha Ridge Press, 2001.

Notes on the State of Virginia. Jefferson, Thomas. W.W. Norton & Company, 1998.

Roadside Geology of Virginia. Frye, Keith. Mountain Press Publishing Company, 2003.

Shenandoah National Park: An Interpretive Guide. Conners, James A. The McDonald & Woodward Publishing Company, 1988.

Virginia: A Guide to Backcountry Travel & Adventure. Bannon, James. Out There Press, 1997.

INDEX

NOTES

SEX AND WORLD PEACE

SEX AND WORLD PEACE

Valerie M. Hudson

Bonnie Ballif-Spanvill

Mary Caprioli

Chad F. Emmett

COLUMBIA UNIVERSITY PRESS   NEW YORK

To Hope Rose and Eve Lily: May your lives be full of joy, confidence, meaning—and action!
To Zakia Zaki and Fawziya Ammodi: We are impoverished by your passage from our world. (D&C 123:13–15)

—*VMH*

To my daughters, whose strength and wisdom astound me.

—*BBS*

To my wife, Laura Chapin, for always believing in me.

—*MC*

To my mother, Norda; my wife, Marie; and my daughter, Sarah. Their goodness inspires me.

—*CFE*

CONTENTS

LIST OF MAPS, FIGURES, AND TABLES

Maps

Figure

Tables

PREFACE AND ACKNOWLEDGMENTS

THE TEAM OF AUTHORS for this book is multidisciplinary, and this is reflected in the text. We have two political scientists who specialize in international relations (Hudson and Caprioli), one geographer who specializes in the study of Islamic societies (Emmett), and one psychologist who specializes in the relationships between socialization, gender, and peace (Ballif-Spanvill). These interests manifest themselves in the literature and examples cited in the book. For example, some of our most detailed micro-analyses are of Islamic nations. This emphasis reflects the in-depth knowledge of the circumstances of these nations held by Emmett. Similarly, the socialization examples are drawn primarily from the psychological literature, and not from political science, reflecting the expertise of Ballif-Spanvill. We believe that this diversity of background and professional training enriches the manuscript.

This book would not exist without the goodwill and hard work of many individuals.

First, we would like to thank the WomanStats coders past and present, including first and foremost our director of operations, S. Matthew Stearmer, without whom the project could not have accomplished what it has thus far. We would also like to thank Jana Pope Badger, Brooke Greer, Thelma Young, Jo Cozzens, Rachel Ligairi, Amy Stevenson, Julie Johnson, Evis Farka, Meg Wilkinson, Becca Hall, Hope Buckman, Tania de Oliveira, Joanna London, Dan Phelps, Melissa Paredes, Leah Raynes, Mary Ann Tanner, Ashley Custer, Emily Pomeroy, Casey Fowles Cox, Nichola Taylor, Katie Phelps, Jason Anderson, V. Matt Krebs, Meghan Foster Raynes, Sarah Roessler, Colleen Johnson, Julianne Parker, Amalia Smith, Margy Hannay Elliott, Douglas Melvin Hansen, Carl Brinton, Laura Summers, Becca Nielsen, Patricia Campbell, Charla Finnigan, Autumn Smith Begay, Lindsey Hulet, Diane

SEX AND WORLD PEACE

1

ROOTS OF NATIONAL AND INTERNATIONAL RELATIONS

When society requires to be rebuilt, there is no use in attempting to rebuild it on the old plan. No great improvements in the lot of mankind are possible until a great change takes place in the fundamental constitution of their modes of thought.

—JOHN STUART MILL

OUR ANALYTICAL MINDS rarely tend toward a holistic view of complex systems, such as national and international relations. For example, take a moment and picture a tree. What do you see? Perhaps you envision a tall tree with many leaves and a big straight trunk with long branches. Do you think about the root system that is sometimes larger than the part of the tree aboveground—the roots that keep the tree alive? What alternatives would you have to heal sick trees or to grow new trees if you never considered the roots? We rarely consider the whole picture, and Mill is right that our own modes of thought are the key to effective and positive change. In this book we ask that you consider the whole picture when examining the world of states and international society. Although often overlooked, sex and gender play a big role in world affairs. By overlooking sex and gender, we limit the policy alternatives that we see in the quest to find solutions to world problems.

In this chapter, which is oriented to undergraduates in international relations (IR) classes, we introduce some of the theories you have been taught about national and international relations and then show you the "roots" of them. We also examine some foundational definitions and concepts that may help us begin to see the roots more clearly. The point is to see the entire tree—not just the part aboveground and not just the roots.

You were taught that a sustainable population meant population control, but were you told that empowering women will naturally restore the population balance? Slowing population growth does not necessarily entail population control—the restriction of the number of children women are allowed to bear. The best approach is to support reproductive freedom for women. With reproductive freedom, women tend to have fewer children. Population

paid labor. Interestingly, those states that invest in their women—for example, ensuring that girls are educated to an equal level with that of boys—are more likely to be wealthy, to be stable, and to be democratic. So taking a gendered perspective allows us to realize that foreign aid to poor states isn't enough to change the underlying inequality that leads to poor economic growth, instability, and autocracy. Policies must target societal norms of gendered inequality and violence that prevent the state from achieving the prosperity, stability, and political freedom its citizens crave.

You were taught that the security of the state rests on power (getting it, keeping it, and displaying it), but were you told that norms of equality create a more sure security for the state? What makes a state safer—power or gender equality? The answer may surprise you: both make a state more secure. Those states that foster gender equality through laws and enforce those laws are less likely to go to war. They are less likely to use force first when in conflict. They are less likely to get involved in violent crises. Once again, a gender-neutral perspective leads you to focus on military might, whereas a gendered perspective highlights the importance of gender equality to facilitate state security.

You were taught that states go to war over oil and scarce resources, but were you told that the roots of violence are even more micro-level than that? States do go to war over oil and scarce resources, among other things, but they are more likely to do so if the society has norms of violence rooted in gender inequality. Violence becomes an acceptable option when women are not considered equals. Here, too, you will find that a gendered perspective leads to different conclusions about international affairs. Oil and scarce resources are a source of conflict, but they do not necessarily lead to war. Those societies that have gender equality are less likely to resort to warfare to meet their resource needs.

You were taught that the clash of civilizations is based on ethnopolitical differences, but did you know that the real clash of civilizations may instead be based on gender beliefs? Samuel Huntington argues that people's cultural and religious identities will be the primary source of conflict in our world; in his view, the fault lines between civilizations will be the battle lines of the future. It would appear, however, that the battle lines of the future are more likely to be found between those states that treat women equally and those states that are fraught with gender inequality. The important cultural distinction is actually between societies that have greater gender equality and those that foster an environment of gender inequality and gender violence. As stated above, societies that are more gender-equal are less likely to go to war,

obvious to see the roots that give rise to the phenomena discussed. Policymakers trying to find solutions to problems are quick to dismiss women as important actors—or do not think about women at all. Yet, as we have shown, it is imperative to take a gendered perspective to understand international issues.

In this book we take a micro-level approach to understanding international relations. We argue that gender inequality is a form of violence that creates a generalized context of violence and exploitation at the societal level. These norms of violence have an impact on everything from population growth to economics and regime type. In IR theory, we assume that our theoretical assumptions, such as the democratic peace thesis, are gender neutral. These assumptions, however, clearly take a male-centric view. We want you to see the whole picture—the tree and the roots—and to experience an approach to understanding that does not exclude but rather embraces a female perspective. It is this gendered approach that is often ignored and might be compared with the roots of the tree. In this book we will make the case that the treatment of women is an unseen foundation for many of the phenomena we see as important in international affairs.

Sex and World Peace offers three major contributions: two of them analytical and one normative. First, we hold that gender inequality, in all of its many manifestations, is a form of violence—no matter how invisible or normalized that violence may be. This gender-based violence not only destroys homes but, we argue, also significantly affects politics and security at both the national and the international levels. This linkage—empirical as well as theoretical—between gender inequality and national and international security is a new approach that has seldom if ever been considered within the discipline of international relations (and other disciplines as well). In a major shift from the conventional understanding, we suggest that efforts to establish greater peace and security throughout the world might be made more effective by also addressing the violence and exploitation that occur in personal relationships between the two halves of humanity, men and women.

A second contribution of this book is to suggest that security studies must include an account of women's security in order to fully address phenomena at the state and system levels. We hope a consideration of the situation of women will become as central to the discussion of world security as power, democracy, religion, culture, resources, and economic growth currently are. We hope that by the time you finish reading this volume, you will consider it quite odd that something so basic and so essential to peace and security is only now beginning to be recognized as such.

sameness or identity. Men and women do not have to be the same to be equal. One can have equality in the context of difference. Therefore, our definition of "inequality" does not denote difference per se; rather it refers to the subordination of one who is different.

FOUNDATIONAL CONCEPTS

WOMEN AS BOUNDARIES OF THE GROUP

Jan Jindy Pettman, extending the work of Nira Yuval-Davis, has called women the boundaries of their nations.[2] What she means by this phrase is that women physically and culturally reproduce their group. While women who are not of the group may physically reproduce it, they will be inadequate cultural reproducers. Only in-group women can play both roles for the group and effectively ensure its survival.

As a result, the capture through force or seduction of women from one group by men of another is not simply a personal issue; it is a group issue. This may be codified in law. For example, take the case of a Lebanese Christian man who married a Muslim woman of the United Arab Emirates and did not convert to Islam: the government of the UAE convicted him of violating Islamic marriage laws and sentenced him to one year in jail and thirty-nine lashes for this offense against the group.[3] Similarly, women in many societies still possess only conditional citizenship, which they may not be able to confer upon their children. A woman's citizenship will be inferred from her father before she is married, and inferred from her husband after she is married. If he is from another country, she may lose her home country citizenship altogether, and her children will be considered citizens of the father's country. In cases where a woman has children out of wedlock with a man from another country, her children may actually end up entirely stateless (see WomanStats variables CLCW and CLCC).[4]

Because of the unique position of in-group women in the group's survival, the group will aim to protect the women from capture by other groups. Indeed, this is one of the reasons why the symbol of a nation is often personified as a woman, in order to elicit these deep feelings of protection. A woman becomes a "protectee" of the men of the group, especially those in her own family. However, as V. Spike Peterson has noted, over time this "protection" begins to elide into "control" and "possession."[5] "Protecting" a woman may

This emphasis on physical purity, where even the suggestion of impurity can ruin a girl, or even destroy a girl, has many far-reaching consequences for women. A girl may be withdrawn from school as soon as she hits puberty, for her sexuality cannot be assured in a context where she may have to walk long distances to school or have a male teacher. A girl may even be married well before puberty—sometimes at seven or eight years of age—to avoid any possibility that her reputation may be destroyed first. Or worse may occur, as in one horrific 2005 case in Pakistan:

Nazir Ahmed appears calm and unrepentant as he recounts how he slit the throats of his three young daughters and their 25-year old stepsister to salvage his family's "honor"—a crime that shocked Pakistan. . . . Ahmed's actions—witnessed by his wife Rehmat Bibi as she cradled their 3 month-old baby son—happened Friday night at their home in the cotton-growing village of Gago Mandi in eastern Punjab province. . . . Bibi recounted how she was woken by a shriek as Ahmed put his hand to the mouth of his stepdaughter Muqadas and cut her throat with a machete. Bibi looked help-lessly on from the corner of the room as he then killed the three girls— Bano, 8, Sumaira, 7, and Humaira, 4—pausing between the slayings to brandish the bloodstained knife at his wife, warning her not to intervene or raise alarm. . . . The next morning, Ahmed was arrested. Speaking to AP in the back of police pickup truck late Tuesday as he was shifted to a prison in the city of Multan, Ahmed showed no contrition. Appearing disheveled but composed, he said he killed Muqadas because she had committed adultery, and his daughters because he didn't want them to do the same when they grew up.

"I thought the younger girls would do what their eldest sister had done, so they should be eliminated," he said, his hands cuffed, his face unshaven. "We are poor people and we have nothing else to protect but our honor." Despite Ahmed's contention that Muqadas had committed adultery—a claim made by her husband—the rights commission reported that accord-ing to local people, Muqadas had fled her husband because he had abused her and forced her to work in a brick-making factory.[10]

From Ahmed's perspective, his own little daughters were an intolerable burden to him, requiring superhuman vigilance. With his honor destroyed by something he could not control—though probably something that had never even occurred—he could not imagine continuing as the father of any

trary, men may be rewarded by their culture for promiscuous behavior. In the age of AIDS, encouraging males to be promiscuous may have deadly consequences not only for men but for women as well, as we will discuss in a later section.

PATRILOCALITY

Another important concept that we must understand in order to see the world through gendered lenses is that of patrilocality. Virtually all traditional cultures remain patrilocal, which simply means that brides relocate to the home of the groom's family upon marriage. Western societies, too, until very recently, were almost always patrilocal. Patrilocality ensures patrilineal inheritance, and patriline claim on all children produced by sons. It also ensures that all men of the clan are kin, mitigating in-group conflict. However, the family psychology produced by patrilocality may have a devastating effect on women and girls. Given concerns over the genetic consequences of inbreeding,[12] girls may find themselves married to grooms who live a substantial distance away from their natal family. Furthermore, as noted above, girls may be married off quite young, for reasons of honor. In such a context, natal families may live with their daughters for only ten to fifteen years and may possibly rarely or never see them again after marriage. In addition, the daughter's children are members of the groom's family, not her natal family.

For all of these reasons, a girl may be viewed as a "houseguest" in her own family. Proverbs testifying to the fact that daughters are not truly members of their natal family abound: "A daughter is a thief." "Raising a daughter is like watering a plant in another man's garden." A girl may come to feel profoundly alienated from her birth family, a feeling that may be reinforced by differential feeding practices and differential access to health care, education, and other resources. Her brothers may eat more, may be taken to doctors, may be encouraged to continue with schooling, and may be excused from chores to do homework. She may notice that she, as a daughter, apparently does not merit this investment from the family, and may draw some natural conclusions from that fact. Boys will draw natural conclusions as well, and will reproduce the same behaviors in their own families.

However, when a girl is married and moves to her husband's family's abode, she will find, in similar fashion, that his family does not consider her a member either. She is an outsider who will never be listed in her husband's genealogy (and will most likely not be listed in her natal family's genealogy).

a sign that a woman is considered a burden and that a groom and his family must be compensated for accepting this burden from the bride's family. This intensifies son preference, for the birth of a daughter may consign a family to bankruptcy when the time comes to pay her dowry. Indeed, signs in India proclaiming, "Better 500 Rupees Now Than 50,000 Rupees Later" are posted to point out in clear economic terms why sex-selective abortion of female fetuses is desirable.[16] If women are commodities akin to livestock, then one can cull them, if necessary, to achieve one's economic ends, such as the avoidance of dowry, or to seek the birth of a son to provide social security in old age. (More on that in a later section.)

In addition, the family of the groom may pressure the bride's family for additional dowry even after the wedding. Girls may be beaten or mutilated to get her family to pay more; if none is forthcoming, the girl may be burned to death in a suspicious "kitchen fire." This frees the groom's family to keep the first dowry (since the husband was widowed, not divorced, and so is not expected to return the dowry) and then to seek a second dowry from the family of another girl. While such practices are by no means attendant in the majority of Indian marriages, they are widespread enough that the Indian government now holds the groom and his immediate family guilty until proven innocent if a young bride dies by household fire.[17]

Of course, we do not see only the wife-as-commodity situation in our world; we also see the female-body-as-commodity. The selling of women's bodies through prostitution, sex trafficking, sex tourism, mail-order brides, militarized prostitution, and even open chattel markets for women and girls in some nations demonstrates that a woman may be bought, sold, and enslaved simply as a set of orifices, with no other meaning or value to her very existence. Indeed, in keeping with a myth prevalent in several countries, that sex with a virgin cures AIDS, women's bodies are "used" in a horrifying way: according to Betty Makoni of the Girl Child Network in Zimbabwe, "The youngest girl I ever came across was a day-old baby who was raped."[18] Trafficked girls who grow too ill due to the AIDS contracted from their users are simply thrown out on the streets to die.

Also left to die are millions of women who are injured or die in pregnancy and childbirth, simply because the meager resources that would be necessary to save their lives are not allocated. Nicholas Kristof and Sheryl WuDunn tell the heartbreaking stories of Mahabouba and Prudence. Mahabouba, of Ethiopia, was sold to a sixty-year-old man when she was a young teenager and had her first stillbirth at fourteen because of obstructed labor resulting in a major

Feminist economists have rightly pointed out that capitalism could not even exist if women did not perform these labors with little or no remuneration.[24] Apparently, in the thinking of most economists, women are like air and water, to be used for free. And economists label women who perform these labors as "non-productive," even though the societies and economies of the world would grind to a halt if all of those "unproductive" women ceased their labors tomorrow.

Capitalism is, in a sense, parasitical upon the free labor, productive and reproductive, that women perform to keep humanity alive through time. Yet the ones on whom our very lives depend are the same ones forced to work without a safety net. Because women are "economically inactive," their caring work means they are largely excluded from social benefits such as health insurance, pensions, and Social Security—except as a woman is joined to an "economically productive" spouse. In the United States, the largest risk factor for poverty in old age is to have ever given birth to a child—that is, to be a mother.[25]

A ROAD MAP OF THIS VOLUME

With these foundational concepts in place, we are prepared to move forward. Chapter 2 lifts the veil on the invisibility of women's reality in our discussion of national and international relations. We argue that the treatment of women—what is happening in intimate interpersonal relationships between men and women—creates a context in which violence and exploitation seem natural. We show how women are disadvantaged by these norms, what wounds are thereby created, and how prevalent such practices are. More fundamentally, we look at why this inequality is invisible, what harm results, and how inequality is maintained through cultural acceptance.

In chapter 3, we provide evidence of the prevalence of inequality and describe the conditions of women. We describe in detail the situation of women across the nations of the world today. We then offer theoretical explanations and empirical evidence concerning the origins of the prevalent social structures favoring men. We explore the impact of those structures on the treatment of women, as well as the diffusion of norms of violence and exploitation throughout society.

Chapter 4 links the micro-level explanations discussed in chapters 2 and 3 to the macro or state level. We empirically demonstrate the linkage between sex and world peace and discuss the need to alter definitions of peace,

2

WHAT IS THERE TO SEE, AND WHY AREN'T WE SEEING IT?

IN THIS CHAPTER we examine how the foundational concepts just surveyed, such as honor and shame, patrilocality, and the devaluation of women's labor, play out in the lives of real women and girls. We argue that what is happening at the most intimate levels can be viewed as a microcosm or a mirror of the larger society—and can provide a way for us to see how violence against women within a society becomes not only pervasive but also "normal." Our contention is that what is considered normal becomes invisible to our eyes, paralyzing us from making needed changes.

THE "LITTLE" THINGS: GENDERED MICROAGGRESSION

The concept of microaggression against women is one worth defining. Gendered microaggression is composed of all those many choices and acts in the routine of day-to-day existence that harm, subordinate, exploit, and disrespect women. These "little" things, experienced day after day, year after year, ground the society in gender inequality and all of its sequelae. Given that gendered microaggression becomes entrenched in daily living, these pernicious norms are the air breathed in by children of both sexes, and they become as natural and invisible to that next generation as air itself. What is viewed as normal is not only invisible but becomes something that is not spoken about either. Silence, often self-imposed, is the sturdy ally of gendered microaggression.

Worse, gendered microaggression may warp women themselves to not only accept violence against them but perpetuate it. Women may be co-opted into

women. We turn now to a discussion of the types of wounds women suffer as a result of such aggression.

While each specific act of gendered microaggression may seem inconsequential to human society, the cumulative impact of millions of acts of microaggression against women is enormous and, as we shall continue to argue, is one of the taproots of violence at all levels, including the international. We proceed by identifying three key wounds inflicted by microaggression against women in human society: (1) lack of bodily integrity and physical security, (2) lack of equity in family law, and (3) lack of parity in the councils of human decision making. We will rely principally on the voices of others to share examples of these wounds.

THE FIRST WOUND: LACK OF BODILY INTEGRITY AND PHYSICAL SECURITY

THE CRUELEST BLOWS: PHYSICAL AND SEXUAL ASSAULT

Sabrija Gerovic was a Bosnian Muslim woman with two children, four-year-old Samira and three-month-old Amira. Early in 1993, during the Bosnian war, she and her children were forced into a truck and driven to a house in Pilnica, where she found herself placed with many other women, Muslims like herself. Her captors were Serb soldiers, *chetniks*.

In the next room were the women aged 15 to 19. "Every night they were taking the girls out."

That night two men came into the room and took her daughter Samira. "She was gone for 24 hours, at midnight the next night a man came in and told me to come and take my child. I went into a room. It was empty and there was only a table.

"They told me to take off my clothes and I was completely naked and there were seven of them. Then they all raped me. They had been drinking but only two were really drunk. One of them was biting at my breast." She pulls back the soiled cream lapels of her shabby navy toweling dressing gown and points to the purple puncture marks all around her left breast. "Here is where he bit me," she said.

"There was a curtain across the room and when they had finished they said: 'Go and get your baby.' I went behind the curtain and [my 4 year old

He made small talk in the lobby, pleasant and unthreatening, so she got into the elevator with him.

And then . . . The man who chatted up, then beat [this woman] did his considerable damage in under 10 minutes.[5]

A horrifying new type of assault against women and girls has even been developed in our modern twenty-first century: acid attacks. For reasons ranging from opposition to a girl's desire to attend school or to her mode of dress, to revenge against a woman's refusal to have sex with or to marry a man, women may be attacked by having hydrochloric or sulfuric acid thrown into their faces. The melting of the face and destruction of the eyes that result take violence against women to a new low:

One morning two months ago [in Afghanistan], Shamsia Husseini and her sister were walking through the muddy streets to the local girls school when a man pulled alongside them on a motorcycle and posed what seemed like an ordinary question

"Are you going to school?"

Then the man pulled Shamsia's burqa from her head and sprayed her face with burning acid. Scars, jagged and discolored, now spread across Shamsia's eyelids and most of her left cheek. These days, her vision goes blurry, making it hard for her to read. . . . [I]n the months before the attack, the Taliban had moved into the Mirwais area and the rest of Kandahar's outskirts. As they did, posters began appearing in local mosques.

"Don't Let Your Daughters Go to School," one of them said.[6]

Is such brutality against women perpetrated only by depraved strangers, then, in or out of war? You know the answer to that question. The answer is "no." The war zone for women extends into the fabric of their daily peacetime lives, a realization that makes us ask sincerely, "Is there ever a true peacetime for women?" All over our world, those most likely to physically injure women are men they love or have loved: husbands, boyfriends, ex-husbands, ex-boyfriends, fathers, brothers. The FBI reports that in single-perpetrator/single-victim homicides, 89 percent of male victims were killed by males, and 90 percent of female victims were killed by males. One-quarter of female homicides are committed by husbands or boyfriends, while 3 percent of male murders are committed by wives or girlfriends. Later studies suggest the 25 percent figure may be too low and that a more in-depth investigation shows

If I am really nervous, I say the cab company's name and the driver's name into the phone. I do this even if there is nobody on the other end of the line.

- When I leave the library or metro stop late at night, I put my keys in my fist, with the points of the keys sticking out between my fingers.
- If the elevator door opens, and I see a man in there and he doesn't get out, unless there are a lot of people around, I don't get into the elevator.
- If I have to drive home alone at night, I lock every door from the inside.
- I make sure I do not look into men's eyes when I walk down the street.
- I would never go hiking or camping by myself.
- If I am in an enclosed space with strangers, I make sure I identify a second way out.
- I find my heart beating wildly when I have to park underground, especially after dark.
- My mom made me take a self-defense class when I was in high school.

Do the answers differ by sex in your classroom or circle of acquaintances? If you are a man, you need to know that the world the women around you live in is not the same as your world. If you are a woman, have you ever stopped to consider just how constrained your life is because of concerns for your personal safety, compared to the life of the young man next to you? This is the first wound.

IT'S NOT SEXY: SEXUAL HARM

This first wound is not confined to the physical assault that we associate with murder, rape, and beatings. The lack of bodily integrity that we are referring to when we speak of "the first wound" is also closely associated with sex itself.

In a way that is not true for men, sex can be deadly for women. What is a moment's pastime for a man may well result in the death of a woman less than a year later. In Sierra Leone, the lifetime chance of a woman dying incidental to pregnancy is one in eight.[12] That's akin to taking an eight-chambered revolver, putting one bullet it, spinning the chamber, and pointing it at your head every time you have sex. Is that what men are thinking of when they have sex? That is certainly what women in Sierra Leone think about when their husbands want sex. They think about the possibility that they may die and leave their children motherless, which in most poor countries is a death

anyplace, anywhere. Refusal went with punishment. I was a complete tyrant in my home.

The women's focus group concurred: "I was only a sex machine for [my husband]. He used me as he wished. I could not argue with him or refuse him sex."

Lack of bodily integrity in sex, of course, results in lack of control over fertility: "Family planning was not a topic ever discussed. It was men who decided how many children and when. Women were just 'baby producing machines.'"

Most people do not know that the United Nations produced a document in 1995 that asserts that women have the right to say no to sex, even if they are married. "The human rights of women include their right to have control over and decide freely and responsibly on matters related to their sexuality, including sexual and reproductive health, free of coercion, discrimination and violence."[17] To suggest that a married woman has the right to say no to sex is, in our opinion, one of the most important breakthroughs in the entire history of human rights. But this international right continues to be virtually unknown by either women or men.

Of course, in the age of AIDS, the right for married women to say no to sex is an important element of self-preservation. Due to the pervasiveness of double standards of marital fidelity throughout the world, where all men, even married men, are encouraged to be promiscuous as a testament to their manhood and where women may be killed even upon unfounded suspicion of sexual relations outside of marriage, a woman's assassin is often her husband, who brings home AIDS to her after visiting prostitutes. (In addition, he may kill more than one wife if the society sanctions polygamy, and may kill the children he sires by giving AIDS to their mother and through the mother to the children.) And, of course, the prostitutes themselves are assassinated by the promiscuous men who bring them AIDS. And, as we have noted earlier, even little girls may be assassinated by men who believe that having sex with a pure child will cleanse them of their AIDS. Women in these societies cannot negotiate the terms upon which they will have sex. They cannot "force" a man to wear a condom. Catherine Maternowska recounts this conversation she had with a truck-stop prostitute in Swaziland:

I met eyes with a 16-year-old named Mbali. She was thin, with close-cropped hair and a beautiful smile. I offered her a packet of crackers, which she

peatedly in an effort to stretch the scar tissue sufficiently for intercourse. In some traditions, the woman must be stitched up again upon becoming pregnant, and then cut open for childbirth. Impaction of the baby's head in the birth canal is common in infibulated women, significantly heightening the risk of stillbirth and maternal death. Vesico-vaginal fistulae, where childbirth opens a passage between a woman's anus and/or her urethra and her vagina, producing an unstoppable flow of urine and feces through the vagina, are a common consequence, and women are almost always divorced and abandoned if a fistula results.

THE SIMPLE FACTS OF LIVING ARE NOT SO SIMPLE FOR WOMEN

Normal daily biological functions may be compromised in other, nonsurgical ways for women. In many areas of the world where indoor plumbing and sanitation are not available, women are able to use field latrines only at dawn and at dusk to avoid harassment and immodesty. They are expected to hold in their urine and feces during the rest of the day, and may be unable to meet their sanitation needs during menstruation.[19] One informant from Kenya told of women having to urinate and defecate in bags during the day, and then having to go out at night and throw the bags as far as they could into the fields. Girls' schooling may become sporadic if there are not adequate facilities for the girls to manage their menstruation at school, and some families may simply take a girl out of school once she begins to menstruate.

Even the basic matter of food may be compromised by gender. The World Bank reports that two-thirds of the most severely malnourished children in India are female.[20] That phenomenon is certainly not restricted to India, and in many regions girls eat last in the household, as this aid worker in Africa notes:

I flew to Kapoeta in southern Sudan. The region was in the midst of a famine; 250,000 people had already starved to death. As is common in Africa, when we landed on the dusty runway families came from miles around to see who had arrived. They knew we were from an aid organization, so mothers held up their emaciated children to show us how much they needed our help. It didn't take me long to notice the children's distended stomachs—a sure sign of malnutrition. But it was several minutes before I realized that in this sea of humanity, the mothers were only holding up sons; there were no daughters. In the familial hierarchy, girls were the last to be fed and the first to die. By the time we arrived, they were dead.[21]

resources preferentially allocated to males. Still other practices that are an expression of physical and sexual dominance of men over women, such as infibulation, chastity belts, droit de seigneur, and gender-based dress codes that inhibit the mobility of women, are also understandable in this light. The convergence in family law systems, expansively defined, through time and space leads us to the conclusion that the formation of family law is at least in part due to dominant men in all cultures having originally created family law through their political power, and having created it in the image of male reproductive interests as shaped by our evolutionary heritage. Baldly put, dominance over females by males is at the foundation of historical family law because of our common evolutionary legacy.

IT SHOULD BE THE HAPPIEST DAY OF THEIR LIVES: MARRIAGE TRAGEDIES

Each inequitable plank in family law fuels tragedy. For example, in many traditional societies, age of consent for girls may be as young as seven or eight. Given the burden of protecting a girl's virginity in honor/shame cultures, girls are typically married off at the onset of puberty, or immediately before. True consent of the bride in marriage, then, is impossible. The marriage has been arranged by her father or her nearest male relative and males from the groom's family. She has probably never met her husband before her wedding. She knows nothing about sex. But her groom is, on average, at least a decade older than she is. Her wedding night, predictably, amounts to child rape, as this memoir by a child bride in Egypt attests. She was thirteen when she was married to her twenty-five-year-old cousin:

> They held my legs apart. One of them held me firmly from behind. One woman gave my groom a clean, white gauze to wrap around his finger. He knew what to do and seemed pleased by my ignorance. . . . He inserted his finger into me, and I screamed. He did this a couple of times until he drew blood. Then he took me and threw me on the bed. I was limp. They gave me a glass of sugar water to revive me. . . . When this was done, each one went her way, and I was alone with him. He closed the door behind him. Suddenly I saw that he was undressed. He has taken off his underpants. I have drawn myself up into a ball on the bed. I was cowering like a fly against the wall. . . . Suddenly I felt myself being moved. He carried me back to the bed and was on top of me . . . I screamed . . . I said no. I was afraid. . . . I

through an e-mail message or an SMS text message. Men need not even register these divorces, or have a court certify them. On the other hand, a Muslim
woman in India would have to prove—in court—one of a set of permissible
conditions for women to divorce, which include insanity or desertion for a
period of at least four years. In other cultures, the permissible reasons may
include male infertility, the husband being in jail due to criminal activity, the
husband bringing another woman into the marital bed, or the husband having AIDS. In short, there is but a small set of legally justifiable reasons for a
woman to divorce, whereas a man may divorce his wife because she put too
much salt on his dinner.[28] Alimony is very rare under such circumstances, and
the woman may not be able to claim any property or assets from the marriage
except for her bride-price. The woman is expected to return to her birth family to live. In turn, her family is usually hard-pressed to support their returning
daughter, and they feel deep shame because of her divorce. Even in Western
societies, divorce often leaves women and children in a far worse economic
situation, while leaving men with greater resources.[29]

The issue of custody of minor children may be tragically inequitable
as well. In most traditional societies, shared custody after divorce is an unknown concept; rather, custody of minor children may automatically devolve
to the father. In many Islamic societies, for example, the rule of thumb is
that custody of a boy is transferred from mother to father at the time the
child is weaned, usually about three years of age. For girls, the child may be
transferred at a specified time between five years of age and puberty, when
it becomes the father's obligation to contract marriage for her. Indeed, the
father may contract a marriage for his daughter over the disapproval of the
girl's mother. If the mother were to remarry, custody of the children must be
transferred to their father immediately upon that marriage. If a father dies, his
widow may lose custody of her children to the father's nearest kin, especially
the paternal grandparents. Because of custody considerations, women in such
societies often remain in abusive marriages so as to be able to maintain a legal
and ongoing relationship with their children.[30] Such considerations are not
unknown even in Western societies as well, because a father's often greater
economic assets may grant him a superior position in court.

And yet even that may not be enough to enable the mother to protect
her children. In Afghanistan, for example, there have been numerous com-
plaints of girls being sold into marriage to much older men as repayment for
debts contracted by their fathers, even over the objections of their mothers.
"Afghans readily use their daughters to settle debts and assuage disputes. Polygamy is practiced. A man named Mohammed Fazal, 45, [said] that village

for life. But . . . Harun's victim was forced with impunity into becoming his wife, in defiance of the law.[34]

This is a long-standing practice in several regions of the world. For example, in one survey of laws in Latin American countries, it was found that in fifteen of those countries the law exonerates a rapist who offers to marry his victim, and in the case of a gang rape, will exonerate all the other men who raped her as long as one offers marriage. In some countries, the law will exonerate a rapist even if the victim refuses to marry him.[35]

It is in the steppes of Central Asia that the practice of marriage-by-rape, euphemistically called "capture marriage," is most prevalent, however, and increasing in prevalence over time. It is estimated that at least one-third of all brides in Kyrgyzstan are abducted and married against their will, and in some rural villages, up to 80 percent of the women have been subject to this practice. A common saying in this culture is "Every good marriage begins in tears."[36]

Bride kidnapping, also called marriage by abduction or marriage by capture, occurs when a young woman, usually below the age of 25, is typically taken through force or deception by a group of men, including the intended groom. Sometimes the men are people she has met prior to the incident; sometimes they are complete strangers. The men are usually drunk; she is usually alone. She is taken to the home of her principal abductor, the intended groom, where his female relatives use physical force and a variety of forms of psychological coercion to compel her to "agree" to the marriage and submit to having the marriage scarf placed on her head—the sign that she consents to marry her abductor. If the kidnapped woman resists, this process can last for hours or days. Her abductor usually rapes her, sometimes prior to her coerced consent to the marriage to shame her to stay rather than go home disgraced. Rape can also occur following the wedding ceremony.[37]

Kyrgyzstan also has the dubious distinction of being the first former Soviet republic to seek to legalize polygamy. Polygamy is quite common in both the Middle East and Africa. In the Middle East, the number of wives taken may be limited by law (often to four), but in some Islamic societies, men are allowed up to ninety-nine *muta'a* marriages, or temporary marriages in which the woman provides sex to a man for a specified price and for a specified time (which may be counted in hours). In the majority of cultures in sub-

Under these ordinances, a woman who had been raped could be stoned to death for adultery:

The evidence of guilt was there for all to see: a newborn baby in the arms of its mother, a village woman named Zafran Bibi. Her crime: she had been raped. Her sentence: death by stoning. Now Ms. Zafran, who is about 26, is in solitary confinement in a death-row cell in Kohat, a nearby town. The only visitor she is allowed is her baby daughter, now a year old and being cared for by a prison nurse.

Thumping a fat red statute book, the white-bearded judge who convicted her, Anwar Ali Khan, said he had simply followed the letter of the Koran-based law, known as hudood, that mandates punishments.

"The illegitimate child is not disowned by her and therefore is proof of zina," he said, referring to laws that forbid any sexual contact outside marriage. Furthermore, he said, in accusing her brother-in-law of raping her, Ms. Zafran had confessed to her crime.

"The lady stated before this court that, yes, she had committed sexual intercourse, but with the brother of her husband," Judge Khan said. "This left no option to the court but to impose the highest penalty."

The man Ms. Zafran accused, Jamal Khan, was set free without charges. A case against him would have been a waste of the court's time. Under the laws of zina, four male witnesses, all Muslims and all citizens of upright character, must testify to having seen a rape take place. The testimony of women or non-Muslims is not admissible. The victim's accusation also carries little weight; the only significant testimony she can give is an admission of guilt.[41]

Fortunately, the federal court overturned Zafran Bibi's punishment, but only after an intensive campaign in the Pakistani media. While the worst elements of the hudood ordinances have been repealed, there still exists the potential for abuse, including stoning to death for false accusations of adultery.[42]

UNEQUAL BEFORE THE LAW: DOUBLE STANDARDS

These cases illustrate also that the testimony of a woman in court may not hold as much weight as the testimony of a man in court. Indeed, in certain conservative Islamic societies, the testimony of a woman is worth exactly half

In an unusually protracted and closely watched case, the Obama adminis-
tration has recommended political asylum for a Guatemalan woman flee-
ing horrific abuse by her husband, the strongest signal yet that the admin-
istration is open to a variety of asylum claims from foreign women facing
domestic abuse.

The large legal question in the case is whether women who suffer domestic abuse are part of a "particular social group" that has faced persecu-
tion, one criteria for asylum claims. In a separate asylum case in April,
the Department of Homeland Security pointed to some specific ways that
battered women could meet this standard.

In a recent filing, Ms. Alvarado's lawyers argued that her circumstances
met the requirements that the department had outlined in April. Now the
department has agreed, in practice making the case a model for other asylum claims.

In a declaration filed recently to bolster Ms. Alvarado's argument that
she was part of a persecuted group in Guatemala, an expert witness, Claudia
Paz y Paz Bailey, reported that more than 4,000 women had been killed
violently there in the last decade. These killings, only 2 percent of which
have been solved, were so frequent that they earned their own legal term,
"femicide," said Ms. Paz y Paz Bailey, a Guatemalan lawyer. In 2008 Guatemala enacted a law establishing special sanctions for the crime.

"Many times," she said, violence against Guatemalan women "is not
even identified as violence, is not perceived as strange or unusual."[47]

A legal system may also defer to other harmful customs concerning women.
In some societies, daughters and wives may by law inherit less than the male
relatives of a deceased person, putting them at greater risk for poverty. In other
societies, widows and their children may actually be inherited as property by
the nearest male relative, usually a brother, of a deceased man. Widow inheritance and another customary law, widow cleansing, which requires that
a widow have sex with some chosen, often marginalized man in her community in order that her husband's spirit not haunt the community, puts these
women at high risk of AIDS infection, in addition to all of the tragedy of
nonconsensual sexual relations. In other communities, the family of the dead
man has the right to evict his widow and children from the property, which
is inherited by his patriline. This has led, in both India and Africa, to a vast
number of AIDS widows and orphans being cast into the street as a result of
the epidemic.[48]

the household. Just as men ruled their households with absolute power, even over the life and death of the members of the household, so a king was the paterfamilias of his nation, with equivalent power over its citizens. Similarly, if the governance of the kingdom began to depart from the accepted template, such as when women began to be perceived as having too much influence on the king, the government would be vulnerable to overthrow by men who saw the regime as "unnatural."[52] Whether we speak of historical figures such as Lady Yang, Marie Antoinette, and Czarina Alexandra or of more modern women who have been perceived as having too much influence on male leaders, such as the twin sister of Shah Reza Pahlavi, the daughter of Boris Yeltsin, or the wife of Bill Clinton, leaders upset the template of male governance at their risk even in the twenty-first century.[53] For example, extremist blog posts from 2007 include statements such as this one concerning Hillary Clinton:

> NOTE: the survival of our Republic is threatened by two things—fundamentalist Islamic terrorists and Hillary Rodham Clinton. President Bush is leading the fight against the terrorists. It is up to those of us who know the real Hillary Clinton to lead the fight against her. We must shine the light of truth on this dangerous woman so that all Americans may know the real Hillary. . . . God help us all if this filthy socialist slut ever takes over America.[54]

> Hillary and her handlers have had Bill doped up and under control for some time now. Remember the few times when he could hardly walk to the podium for a speech. . . . They let him screw whatever he wanted and he was happy while others ran things.[55]

You do not have to be a supporter of Hillary Clinton to believe that something much, much deeper than Clinton herself was being attacked here.

In a way, these deep feelings go back to what a group, a collective, a nation actually is. In evolutionary terms, as we have seen, the fundament of human groups has been the male kin group. Practicing universal exogamy, while women leave the group upon marriage, the men—all kin—stay. The group, in this sense, belongs to the men, and they perceive themselves to be its rightful rulers in many traditional societies. The ancient Greeks opined that women may give birth to babies, but men give birth to nations. Blood sacrifice in birth was viewed as trivial next to blood sacrifice in war, which is

An additional rationale for this exclusion involved the idea that women were insufficiently motivated to act in the national interest, as opposed to the common human interest. This stunning anecdote from a male Cold War physicist, as recounted by Carol Cohn, summarizes the point:

"Several colleagues and I were working on modeling counterforce attack, trying to get realistic estimates of the number of immediate fatalities that would result from different deployments. At one point, we remodeled a particular attack, using slightly different assumptions, and found that instead of there being thirty-six million immediate fatalities, there would only be thirty million. And everybody was sitting around nodding, saying, 'Oh yea, that's great, only thirty million,' when all of a sudden I *heard* what we were saying. And I blurted out, 'Wait, I've just heard how we're talking—Only thirty million! Only thirty million human beings killed instantly?' Silence fell upon the room. Nobody said a word. They didn't even look at me. It was awful. I felt like a woman."[60]

One of us has a personal anecdote in this regard, as a woman looking at this same phenomenon:

I was sitting in the annual American Political Science Association meeting one year during the Cold War. Being a security expert, I was attending panels on that topic. I found myself sitting in on a panel discussing NATO strategy. On the panel were all bright young men in the right color and cut of suits, with glasses and briefcases, and I was the only woman in the room. After the presentations were over, a foreign scholar in the audience rose and asked, "Exactly what is NATO's Follow-On Forces Strategy? I am unfamiliar with that term." One of the bright young men said, "Oh, that's easy to understand. It's a series of swift, penetrating thrusts to the enemy's rear!" Whereupon, yours truly lost it. I started to giggle uncontrollably, could not stop to save my life, and had to leave the room under the stares of my peers. Out in the hall, I realized that I wasn't sure if I should be laughing or crying.

These patriarchal norms of dominance and control as the route to security and peace are deeply flawed, but they still permeate much of human society, even in the twenty-first century. To the extent they do, we will still hear the echo of the ultranationalist Russian politician Vladimir Zhirinovsky, who,

A DEFICIT OF WOMEN, A DEFICIT OF GOOD GOVERNMENT

What differences are noted when women are significantly represented in human government? Researchers are just beginning to uncover the differences, as there historically have been so few nations with significant percentages of women legislators. Political variables at the state level have also been related to the situation of women, most specifically levels of corruption. For example, a study of eighty countries found a negative correlation between indices of corruption and indices of women's social and economic rights.[63] Because a decrease in political corruption increases investment and growth, gender equity thus has additional influence on economic growth.[64] According to an Inter-Parliamentary Union survey of 187 women holding public office in sixty-five countries,[65] women's presence in politics increases the amount of attention given to social welfare, legal protection, and transparency in government and business, and 80 percent of respondents said that women's participation restores trust in government.

Ann Crittenden has authored a serious argument for taking the perspectives of women seriously in public policymaking. She quotes Ann Richards, former governor of Texas, as saying,

"When policy is made in government or in law, when any people whose lives are going to be affected aren't at the table and in on the decisions, the reactions aren't going to be as good. For example, when I was Travis county commissioner in Austin, I had decisions to make about the hospital system. My husband had some strong opinions on the subject, and as he spoke, it dawned on me that he hadn't been in a hospital since he was a child. I'd been in a bunch more times than he had, having four children and a few other things. Now here was a strongly held opinion from someone who'd had essentially no experience being in a hospital. Someone with that experience should be the first person brought in to talk about whatever problems there are. . . . So women's presence, and especially the presence of women with children, is essential when decisions are made about child care, medical care, education, mental health, taxes, war and peace."[66]

Crittenden notes that female legislators will break party ranks on issues that are important to mothers and children, and observes that female Republican legislators often do so. And of course, in 2010, it was Republican senator

As development became more integrated with a gender perspective, other state-level phenomena also began to be seen through a gender lens, with important results. Analysis of the effects of women's education was a natural next step. For example, the World Bank has concluded that low investment in female education reduces a country's overall output. One study found that if South Asia, sub-Saharan Africa, and the Middle East and North Africa had invested earlier in closing gender gaps in education, their income per capita would have increased by 0.5 to 0.9 percent from 1960 to 1992.[75] A study of ninety nations concluded that a 1 percent increase in female to male primary enrollment rates increases GDP growth by 0.012 percent.[76] In addition, the more education a mother has, the lower her children's mortality rates, even after controlling for household income and socioeconomic status.[77] A study conducted in the Philippines concluded that a mother's education was more of a contributing factor to her children's health status than household income,[78] and another cross-national study of sixty-three nations determined that women's education was the single most important factor in levels of malnutrition over a twenty-five-year period.[79]

HALF-BRAINED DECISION MAKING

Economic prosperity and system stability in more-developed countries are also affected by the degree of women's voice. Indeed, the recent global recession has been blamed on women's lack of voice in economic decision making. John Coates and Joseph Herbert, publishing in the *Proceedings of the National Academy of Sciences*, found that testosterone levels correlated significantly with risk taking among stock market traders.[80] Victories on the stock floor led to higher levels of testosterone and higher levels of risk taking. Coates commented, "Male traders simply don't respond rationally."[81]

Over the course of time, natural selection has rewarded men who have certain characteristics with more offspring: among these reproductively successful men are men who form tight bonds with other men, men who resort to physical force to get what they want, men who lack empathy, men who are highly motivated to garner resources with minimum effort, men who are willing to take risks, men who subordinate "others," whether those others be women or strangers.[82] Cooperating with other men in "in-groups" to take resources from "others" with a mix of minimum effort, high risk, and disregard of harm done to others is a skill that men, generally speaking, possess because

Recent research has also shown that when both males and females make decisions together, all participants are more satisfied with the outcome than when decisions are the product of all-male groups.[85] Furthermore, researchers have found that mixed decision-making groups are less accepting of risk than all-male groups, and that non-zero-sum outcomes are more likely.[86] Having more women not only as significant governmental actors but also as significant economic actors may actually be good for business. Real gender equality, including a meaningful sharing of power within society, may thus be a prerequisite for optimal and rational policymaking, whether for households, countries, or the international community.

THE BOYS' WORLD OF ECONOMIC UNREALITY

However, women are systematically excluded from our conventional understanding of the economic system. Think for a moment about the fact that when male economists in the 1930s developed the national system of accounts, they decided that women in their traditional roles as housewives were economically inactive, producing nothing of value to the society. Marilyn Waring explains:

Consider Tendai, a young girl in the Lowveld, in Zimbabwe. Her day starts at 4 a.m., when, to fetch water, she carries a thirty litre tin to a borehole about eleven kilometers from her home. She walks barefoot and is home by 9 a.m. She eats a little and proceeds to fetch firewood until midday. She cleans the utensils from the family's morning meal and sits preparing a lunch of sadza for the family. After lunch and the cleaning of the dishes, she wanders in the hot sun until early evening, fetching wild vegetables for supper before making the evening trip for water. Her day ends at 9 p.m., after she has prepared supper and put her younger brothers and sisters to sleep. Tendai is considered unproductive, unoccupied, and economically inactive. According to the international economic system, Tendai does not work and is not part of the labour-force.

Cathy, a young, middle-class North American housewife, spends her days preparing food, setting the table, serving meals, clearing food and dishes from the table, washing dishes, dressing her children, disciplining children, taking the children to day-care or to school, disposing of garbage, dusting, gathering clothes for washing, doing the laundry, going to the gas station and the supermarket, repairing household items, ironing, keeping

are the future of our societies. Nancy Folbre calls this labor "the invisible heart," playing off the concept of the "invisible hand" of Adam Smith.[93] But while the invisible hand is an inanimate fiction, the invisible hearts belong to real women who are performing real and absolutely necessary labor for the members of the human family—and do so without any valuation of that labor, and without any safety net. At one of the universities at which we teach, Econ 101 introduces the study of economics using a scenario involving two healthy adult men—Robinson Crusoe and Friday—alone on an island, who then end up trading palm fronds and coconuts. If this is the way we introduce young people to thinking about what an economy is, no wonder our economy has serious distortions. We have often daydreamed of beginning an Economics 101 class with this alternative scenario: "There once was a woman, and she had just given birth to a child, and was exhausted, hungry, and losing blood." What kind of economics would be taught if that were the foundational scenario? As Waring remarks concerning the "naively masculine" science of economics,

> What changes might occur in global economic policy and practice if the worth . . . of the majority of [the] human population were *valued*? . . . [T]he satisfaction of basic needs to sustain human society is fundamental to any economic system. By this failure to acknowledge the primacy of reproduction, the male face of economics is fatally flawed. We frequently hear from politicians, theologians, and military leaders that the wealth of a nation is its children. But, apparently, the creators of that wealth deserve no economic visibility for their work. . . . [I]f you have a conceptual problem about the activity of half the human species, you then have a conceptual problem about the whole.[94]

Here we see in microcosm the costs of systematically excluding women from the work of credentialed knowledge creation in our society. Because men created the science of economics—as well as many other sciences—we have a grossly distorted view of the priorities and needs of our society. Unjustified assumptions go unquestioned. Fantasies pass for sophisticated models. Pressing questions go unasked. Alternative answers go unheard. If our departments of economics had a sizable representation of mothers on their faculties, the entire science would be transformed. Consider:

> The changing pattern of layoffs is a portent of the "friction free" economy that many economists aspire to. "It's an economist's wet dream," says Roger Martin, dean of the Rotman School of Management at the University of

women working at the Population Council, and then the Ford Foundation's population office, in the early 1970s. "It's as though women weren't human," she now recalls. Senior professional staff "could walk the corridors and be in meetings and talk about 'users' and 'acceptors' and write about users and acceptors and have absolutely no interest in who these people were." Women were excluded from discussion about contraceptive technology and the ethics of research trials. When Nafis Sadik arrived at UNFPA in 1971, she already had sixteen years of experience as a gynecologist and public health professional, culminating with her nomination as director-general of the Pakistani General Council for Family Planning. But in her new workplace, where she was the only professional woman, "it felt as if I didn't exist." Any substantive suggestions she made "fell on deaf ears." Even in the IPPF, women were underrepresented on the key budget, finance, medical and scientific committees. As for the World Bank, it did not have even one professional woman involved in population programs.

Worse yet was the sexual harassment many women experienced. "The way some women were treated by some of the topmost of the senior leaders was despicable," Germain recalls, "whether it's how they treated their graduate students, or how they behaved at the huge number of conferences . . . specially by Northern men via-a-vis women in foreign countries." One senior official bragged to the author about his escapades at these meetings, including having sex with one woman in a conference room after other participants had left. Asked whether he used protection, he replied, "I let her worry about that . . ."

A number of demographers, including Irene Taeuber, were interested in how women's access to education and paid work was correlated with lower fertility and might therefore bring down birth rates in poor countries. . . . The separation of men and women, the qualitative and quantitative, and the First and Third Worlds, meant that this crucial insight about the relationship between women's education and fertility was overlooked when it came to designing policies and programs. . . . It was not until more professional women won a place in international debates that promoting [women's] education became the solution. . . . [I]t is the emancipation of women, not population control, that has remade humanity.[97]

Again, it is hard not to gasp at the audacity of men attempting to solve population problems while excluding women from the discussion and the policymaking. But as this chapter has shown, the most important problems of our day, whether those be population problems, development problems,

Yet ordinary villagers themselves judged the women as having done a worse job, and so most women were not re-elected. That seemed to result from simple prejudice. Professor Duflo asked villagers to listen to a speech, identical except that it was given by a man in some cases and by a woman in others. Villagers gave the speech much lower marks when it was given by a woman.

Such prejudices can be overridden after voters actually see female leaders in action. While the first ones received dismal evaluations, the second round of female leaders in the villages were rated the same as men. "Exposure reduces prejudice," Professor Duflo suggested.[100]

In surveying this research, it appears that the obstacles to women's having a real voice in the decision-making councils of humanity are large indeed. They may speak, but will they even be heard? If exposure actually does reduce prejudice, we can only hope that through a concerted and purposeful effort by humankind to include women in decision-making councils at all levels of society and in sufficient numbers that their distinctive perspective is supported and not quashed, over time the two halves of humanity may, finally, together guide their world. We have every reason to believe that joint stewardship would produce better results than the exclusion of half of the species from decision making. That such a true sharing of power and voice between men and women is still rare in human society is the third great wound that humanity must address.

We have spoken of what we perceive to be the three wounds caused by gendered microaggression and afflicting women in the house of humanity. The first is the lack of bodily integrity and personal safety for women; the second is the codification of unequal status before the law, especially in personal status and family law, between men and women; and the third is the lack of decision-making parity between men and women in the councils of humanity at all levels, small and great. We now turn to an empirical survey of the incidence and prevalence of these wounds, and we will make initial inquiries into the origins of gender inequality.

MAPPING THE WORLDWIDE SITUATION OF WOMEN

What follows, then, is a series of maps that we hope will better illustrate the varying patterns and the complexities of the situation of women in the countries of the world. These maps are generalizations, and so it is important to remember that the individual lives of women may not correspond to the overall condition of women in the country. Despite all of these caveats, through these maps it will become apparent that there is much work to be done and that some countries are doing better than others.

The scales used in the maps were developed by our project team and coded using the data in the WomanStats Database. These are 5-point ordinal scales, and each ranges from 0 to 4, with 0 being the best condition (often in the text called, somewhat counterintuitively, the "highest" rank) and 4 being the worst condition (often in the text called the "lowest" rank). Some of the scales are multivariate in nature, while others address a single variable. So, for example, our multivariate Physical Security of Women Scale looks at several different variables, such as murder, rape, and so forth. Our Educational Discrepancy Scale, on the other hand, looks specifically at laws, practices, and data concerning secondary education of girls, and so addresses but one cluster of variables. While we will mention the scale descriptions in the text, a fuller description of how each scale was coded can be found in the online WomanStats codebook; http://womanstats.org/CodebookCurrent.html.

PHYSICAL SECURITY OF WOMEN

Our first map, map 1, shows a surprising range and interesting patterns concerning women's physical security. It is based on a multivariate scale, the Physical Security of Women Scale, most recently assessed in 2009, that includes variables for domestic violence, rape, marital rape, and murder (MULTIVAR-SCALE-1 in the WomanStats Database). It examines not only incidence of violence against women but also whether or not there are laws against such practices and whether or not those laws are enforced.

Sadly, no country achieved the highest ranking (0), which would indicate that women are physically secure. To obtain such a ranking a country would have laws against not only murder but also domestic violence, rape, and marital rape; those laws would be enforced; and there would be no taboos or norms against reporting these crimes, which would be rare.

We find some interesting patterns in this mapping. Catholic Ireland and Muslim Tunisia are at the same rank (4) as Hindu India and several Confucian countries (including Taiwan, South Korea, and Singapore). This worst rank also includes several Western European countries—among them Portugal and Switzerland, which were two of the highest ranked on the Physical Security of Women Scale. The general middle ranking of the Middle East in terms of sex ratio is a significant divergence from what we see with the Physical Security of Women Scale. Iceland and four Caribbean countries rank the best, with no noted preference for sons and the most normal sex ratios. In fact, a comparison of the Physical Security of Women map and the Son Preference and Sex Ratio map is perplexing: why is there so little correlation between levels of violence against women as adults and levels of violence against women as neonates?

The average Son Preference and Sex Ratio for all states in 2006 was 2.07 and in 2009 was 2.41, indicating a general, globalized son preference. This in itself is an important characteristic of our current world system that often goes unremarked. Globally, male offspring are valued more highly than female offspring. However, since the average is in the range of 2 on a scale of 0–4, this generalized son preference does not appear to necessarily result in female infanticide or sex-selective abortion in most states. Nevertheless, the comparatively low value ascribed to female life penetrates every aspect of women's daily lives, thus both perpetuating the cycle of gendered violence[1] and resulting in their own diminished sense of self.

As we have noted, Son Preference and Sex Ratio is not necessarily correlated with violent practices against adult women. This highlights the crucial importance of using a multivariate approach to assess the status of women. Just as different cultures vary in the way they perpetuate violence against women, the incidence of such violence varies across the life span from the fetus to the widow. Practices such as female infanticide and passive neglect strike women in their earliest years, whereas practices such as dowry deaths affect young adult women, and other practices such as inheriting of widows or the turning out of widows occur later in life.

TRAFFICKING IN FEMALES

Trafficking in females is inherently an act of violence that assaults women's human rights. The trafficking cluster, from which we create our ordinal

The global average is 1.6 on our scale. Countries where polygyny is legal and where it is more commonly practiced are primarily found in Saharan and sub-Saharan Africa. Interestingly, much of the Islamic world, where the religion allows for up to four wives if they are treated fairly by the husband, generally falls within the middle category of countries where polygyny is either legally constrained or technically legal but practiced in fewer than 5 percent of marriages. There are some Islamic countries that have more prevalent polygyny, among them Saudi Arabia and some of the Gulf States, Yemen, Afghanistan, Morocco, and Turkey.

Over time, increasing numbers of countries have moved from scale point o to scale point 2, as minority, usually immigrant, populations in Western nations continue to practice polygyny. While Western nations have not legalized polygyny per se, many do recognize the polygynous marriages of immigrants from countries where polygyny is legal. Other countries, such as France, insist on "de-cohabitation" of polygynous immigrant families. Given the association in the literature between polygyny and societal instability, it will be interesting to trace these trajectories over time.

INEQUITY IN FAMILY LAW/PRACTICE

As we will see in subsequent chapters, many of the top-down and bottom-up efforts to improve the status of women focus on rectifying inequities in a state's family law, and how that law is practiced on the ground. Our Inequity in Family Law/Practice Scale, most recently scaled in 2011, is a true multivariate scale, examining aspects of family law and practice such as legal age of marriage for girls, issues of female consent in marriage, polygyny, marital rape, inheritance rights of widows, rights of women in divorce, and so forth (map 5).

The eighteen countries where family law/practice is equitable for women are predictably found in Western Europe, plus Canada, New Zealand, and Australia (interestingly, neither the United States nor the United Kingdom made the cutoff; they are both at the next scale point, 1). The criteria of law and practice found in these countries of highest rank include legal age of marriage for women at least eighteen, with most women (more than 50 percent) marrying after that age. Marrying at an age younger than sixteen is virtually unknown in these countries. Polygyny is illegal and extremely rare. Women are free to choose their spouse. Women know their rights to consent and divorce and are free to exercise those rights without fear of reprisal. Marital

2010, ranks countries according to maternal deaths per 100,000 births (map 6). The global average was 2.45 on our 5-point scale ranging from 0–4, meaning that most countries in the world have relatively high maternal mortality rates.

The countries with the lowest maternal mortality rates include, once again, Sweden with the highest ranking with only 2 deaths per 100,000 births. Noteworthy is that among the twenty-two other countries with death rates below 10 per 100,000 are Kuwait and Qatar. Nestled in the second tier (scale point 1) are the United States (17 per 100,000), with Saudi Arabia (23 per 10,000), and Bahrain (28 per 100,000) only slightly behind. The inclusion of four Arab states in these top two tiers might be dismissed by some as only reflective of high GDP per capita, but the fact that these Arab/Islamic countries have built hospitals and clinics and provided an education for female obstetricians and nurses suggests that woman are valued and supported as mothers in these societies.

The soberingly high maternal mortality rates among many African states should be seen as a call to arms by the rest of the world to help women through the vulnerable life stages of pregnancy and birth. It is a true devaluation of women's lives for the state to be indifferent as to whether they live or die as a result of bringing forth the next generation of citizens.

DISCREPANCY IN EDUCATION

Our Discrepancy in Education Scale, most recently scaled in 2010, examines the rates of secondary education among girls and boys, looking specifically at differences in rates of attainment of this level of education, as well as whether there are any legal or cultural restrictions on girls' education at this level (map 7).

The global average for this scale is 1.63, with an average gap of about 4.85 percent between male and female rates of secondary education. There are some clear regional patterns. Western Europe, for the most part, scores very well on this scale (with the exception of Switzerland, which scores very poorly in comparison to its neighbors). Sub-Saharan Africa and South Asia are both regions where the educational attainment of girls is significantly below that of boys, and where, in fact, there may be important barriers, legal or cultural, to girls' education. Other areas are quite diverse. For example, in the Islamic world, we have, on the one hand, nations such as Algeria, Oman, and Libya, which score very well (scale point 1), but also several countries scoring the middle rank of 2, this is a quite counterintuitive finding. Other relatively wealthy industrialized nations come in at an even worse ranking than the United States. Japan, Singapore, and South Korea are in the worst tier of nations (scale point 4) for governmental participation of women.

Anomalies abound in this category. Macedonia is in the best scale rank; Greece is in the next-to-lowest rank. Chile is in the best; Brazil is in the worst. In comparing across scales, we also find some interesting phenomena: South Africa, with one of the lowest rankings on physical security of women, is in the highest rank of nations for governmental participation of women.

Also noteworthy is that the representation of democracies in the worst ranks of the Governmental Participation by Women Scale is higher than expected. As noted previously, nations such as Japan and South Korea, as well as Brazil, all score in the worst rank on the scale. In the next-to-worst rank, we find democracies such as India, Greece, Slovenia, and Hungary.

INTERMINGLING IN PUBLIC IN THE ISLAMIC WORLD

In many of the above maps we can see that even within regions with strong cultural and religious influences, significant differences are apparent. We will now look at two maps and scales dealing with issues concerning women specifically in the Islamic world: the intermingling of women and men in society and required dress codes for women. Both maps show a wide variance in the rankings and belie the view of many a mental map that all women of the Islamic world are subject to the same rigid requirements.[2] Furthermore, given the massive transformation of the Arab world in 2011, that variance may well expand. The first map, showing our assessment of intermingling in public in the Islamic world, most recently evaluated in 2008, addresses the practices of separating men and women in public places and of limiting the movement of women in public when they are not accompanied by a male relative (map 9).[3]

The map shows that most of the Islamic countries do not have legal restrictions on women's freedom of movement within public spaces. Social restrictions, however, are extremely common, and in many instances are just as limiting. The prevalence of patrilocality in the Middle East lends legitimacy to beliefs that a woman is the property of her husband's extended family and therefore does not have the right to travel without permission of a husband or male guardian. Most Islamic countries can be characterized as honor/shame societies, in which the perceived sexual purity of women is a direct reflection

part of the legal code and are enforced by state police. In Saudi Arabia, boys and girls are generally segregated beginning at puberty, and sex segregation is enforced in schools, restaurants, banks, and other public buildings. The labor code prohibits the intermingling of men and women in work settings. Everything a woman does is subject to the approval of a *mahram*, or male relative. Women must have the permission of a male guardian to obtain a passport or travel abroad, and in fact are not even supposed to be out in public without a *mahram*. Additionally, "visible and invisible spatial boundaries also limit women's movement. Mosques, most ministries, public streets, and food stalls (supermarkets not included) are male territory. Furthermore, accommodations that are available for men are always superior to those accessible to women, and public space, such as parks, zoos, museums, [and] libraries."[4] The Saudi Committee for the Promotion of Virtue and the Prevention of Vice is the organization charged with enforcing segregation laws. It is the almost universal enforcement of these laws that separates Iran and Saudi Arabia from neighboring countries that may not have the means or manpower to enforce them. In recent years Saudi Arabia's laws have come under international condemnation as a result of high-profile news events. In 2002 fourteen school-aged girls died in a fire at their school when the virtue and vice police prevented them from leaving the burning building because they did not have *mahram*s to accompany them home, and actually prevented rescue workers from entering the building because unrelated men and women are not supposed to intermingle. And in 2006 a gang-rape victim was sentenced to an unbelievable ninety lashes for being in a taxi with an unrelated man right before her rape.

Laws and the enforcement of laws in the Islamic Republic of Iran are likewise comparably strict. The 1979 Islamic revolution in Iran brought about many changes for the country's women. Coed schools are now banned by the Ministry of Education, and women are required to have a husband's permission to work outside the home. Women are restricted from riding in specific sections of buses and from using the main entrances in public buildings. They are also banned from attending sporting events.

REQUIRED CODES OF DRESS FOR WOMEN IN THE ISLAMIC WORLD

Some societies enforce required dress codes for women; this practice is most prevalent in Islamic societies, taking the form of certain garments and/or veils (map 10, which reflects our most recent assessment, in 2008). Veiling acts

hijab) became popular about fifteen years ago as part of an Islamic revival. Islamist movements in the Gaza Strip began pressuring women to veil in the 1980s. Although Indonesia is a secular nation, there has been a trend toward Islamization and as a result headscarves are now very common.

At the same time, however, Islamization and the spread of fundamentalism are causing political unrest in many other countries. In Kuwait, the use of the *niqab* (covers all of the face but the eyes) has shifted from a distinct dress associated with Bedouin women to a political symbol associated with fundamentalism and has consequently sparked debate between liberals and conservatives in the country. In Libya under Gaddafi, a woman wearing a *niqab* would be suspected of Islamism, and therefore antigovernment activity.

Because many of the secular governments in Islamic countries fear Islamization and the popularity of Islamic fundamentalism, they attempt to enact laws or policies that restrict women's right to wear a veil. This limitation is manifested differently depending on the country. In Libya under Gaddafi schoolteachers were not allowed to wear the *niqab*. As in most central Asian countries, the wearing of a headscarf in official photographs is prohibited in Azerbaijan. Secondary schools in Kyrgyzstan will not allow girls who wear veils to attend school. The Education Ministry in Tajikistan has likewise banned Islamic headscarves at schools and universities. Female students have been expelled from universities in Uzbekistan for wearing Islamic veils. In Egypt (before the revolution of 2011), where 80 percent of women veil, government-sponsored newspapers discouraged the *niqab* and state-run television networks prohibited wearing the veil on air. Morocco has recently removed references to and pictures of veils in its textbooks.

Elsewhere, opposition to veiling is even stronger. In Tunisia (speaking of conditions before the revolution of 2011) it is against the law to wear a *hijab* in public office buildings, and government ministers frequently denounce the wearing of veils as foreign to Tunisia's traditions. The original decree against *hijabs*, which has since been repealed, "led to an oppressive campaign against veiled women in public institutions, in the streets, on public transport and in hospitals. It included violence against the women, the tearing of their clothing and their removal to security centres."[6] In recent years government policies against veiling have led to violent clashes between the police and Islamist rebels. As noted previously, no one yet knows how the uprisings of 2011 will affect dress codes for women.

Turkey, where more than 60 percent of women veil, also has banned wearing veils in schools and universities, and many women have been deprived of

HOW DID MALE-DOMINATED SOCIAL STRUCTURES DEVELOP THROUGHOUT HUMAN CULTURES?

To establish the theoretical linkage between the security of women and the security of states, we synthesize insights from several disciplines, including evolutionary biology and psychology, which provide an account of basic tendencies of human behavior in terms of natural selection; biological, developmental, and social psychology, which provide an account of more proximate causal mechanisms of diffusion in terms of cultural selection through social learning; and social psychology and political sociology, which offer an account of the social diffusion of both naturally selected and culturally selected traits.

EVOLUTIONARY BIOLOGY AND PSYCHOLOGY

Evolutionary biology and psychology have been underutilized by social scientists, leading political scientist Bradley Thayer to comment that "this leads to an artificially limited social science" using assumptions about human behavior that may be "problematic, or fundamentally flawed."[7] Evolutionary theory provides explanations in terms of ultimate cause, not proximate cause, framing the context within which individual creatures strive to increase their fitness (survival and reproductive success). Differential fitness levels, then, drive natural selection: if one survives to reproduce (or if one can facilitate the reproduction of close kin, a concept termed "inclusive fitness"), natural selection will move in the direction of one's genotype. Changes in rates of survival and reproduction among individuals and kin groups will therefore eventually change the genotype of the overall population.

Evolutionary theory suffers from two common misconceptions. The first is that evolutionary predispositions are intractable. No evolutionary theorist believes this. Richard Dawkins explains, "It is perfectly possible to hold that genes exert a statistical influence on human behavior while at the same time believing that this influence can be modified, overridden, or reversed by other influences."[8] The second misconception is that evolutionary theory posits static and essential characteristics for males and females. In debunking this myth, Theodore Kemper notes, "Across the spectrum of the social sciences, the results show that females are not essentially pacific, retiring, unaggressive, lacking in motives and psychological need for power and dominance. While

duction and parental investment in offspring survival.[16] As Archer explains, "the sex showing higher parental investment becomes a limiting resource, the other sex competing for reproductive access."[17] In a similar manner, differences in the reproductive success of males and females further drive competitive processes of sexual selection. Whereas females are not able to mate again immediately after producing offspring, males do not experience any interruption and can therefore move on to mate with other females to increase their reproductive success.

While there are a wide variety of male-female interactions that result in reproduction, one of the most common in nonhuman primates is sexual coercion by the male of the female, according to Smuts. Such coercion lowers males' costs of reproduction, compared to strategies such as assisting females in the care of the young. Such sexually coercive strategies involve not only forced copulation (usually on pain of physical violence), but also infanticide by males of nonrelated offspring of the female with whom he seeks copulation. Smuts explains that the females typically do mate with these males who have killed their infants, thereby reducing the females' reproductive success, in order to receive protection for their future offspring.[18] They may also have little choice in resisting mating with a violent male who could potentially kill the female as well as her infants. Sexual coercion, then, can be effective as a male mating strategy.

Indeed, evolutionary biologist Patricia Adair Gowaty suggests that even sexual dimorphism can be better explained if we place relations between the sexes as the most influential factor in its development: "Female-male competition over control of female reproduction is an untested, viable alternative to the male-male competition explanation for 'males larger' in sexually dimorphic species."[19] Interestingly, Gowaty's own research demonstrates that in contrast to the typical "coy" behavior of females in a typical group setting, when males and females have been reared separately (and thus females have never witnessed male-on-female violence), females do not exhibit "coyness" or choosiness when introduced to the males, suggesting that they have not yet learned to fear male aggression.[20]

The first conflict among humans, then, was the clash of reproductive interests between males and females. This leads Rosser to assert, "Women's oppression is the first, most widespread, and deepest oppression,"[21] and Gowaty to opine, "[S]exist oppression is fundamental to—is 'the root' of—all other systems of oppression."[22] This is why Smuts believes that patriarchy predates agriculture. Smuts concludes that "men use aggression to try to control women,

for status, resources, and females is a universal feature of human societies."[27] Again, male reproductive advantage appears to be the root. Anthropologist Napoleon Chagnon's research into hunter-gatherer societies demonstrates that individual men who are aggressive have a higher status in the village and greater reproductive success.[28] Simply put, "Better fighters tend to have more babies. That's the simple, stupid, selfish logic of sexual selection."[29]

As such fraternal alliances developed, the male dominance hierarchy structure was increasingly selected as a way to dampen male-male competition within the group. Indeed, pair-bonding in human societies may have developed as a social structure to that very end—that is, to produce "male respect of the mating privileges of their allies."[30] With amelioration of in-group conflict among males, such male dominance hierarchies were more effective in coercing women, as well as in facing threats from out-group male coalitions. These male coalitions also formed the foundation for male control of economic resources important for female reproduction. Male hunting parties would control division of game; male raiding parties would control division of spoils. Smuts notes, "[M]en may use their alliances with other men to prevent actions that may benefit the women, but at a cost to the men."[31]

Male dominance hierarchies can, however, become extremely hierarchical, with some men controlling a vastly disproportionate share of the resources and power. Smuts hypothesizes that in such inegalitarian contexts, women will be subject to the most extreme forms of coercion, as the fear of powerful men over "the problem of imperfect monopolization of the mate" increases.[32] Powerful men with greater resources have much more to lose than poor men if their control over women is ineffective, and so they will use their resources and power to ensure that they will not be losers. Smuts suggests, "[T]he degree to which men dominate women and control their sexuality is inextricably intertwined with the degree to which some men dominate others."[33]

This has important ramifications for the development of the political system. In environments where resources are distributed more equitably, males will exhibit less aggressive behavior toward one another. This holds in contemporary studies of violence: "evidence indicates that relative deprivation (as indexed by income inequality) is typically a more powerful predictor of variation in male violence than other socioeconomic measures such as percent below the poverty line or average income."[34]

This increasing male monopoly over the economic resources needed by females for reproduction is not mirrored in nonhuman primates, where

Patriarchy is worldwide and history-wide, and its origins are detectable in the social lives of chimpanzees. It serves the reproductive purposes of the men who maintain the system. Patriarchy comes from biology in the sense that it emerges from men's temperaments, out of their evolutionarily derived efforts to control women and at the same time have solidarity with fellow men in competition against outsiders. . . . Patriarchy has its ultimate origins in male violence.[42]

As we have noted, given the natural selection of sexual dimorphism in humans, violence and coercion are an effective male mating strategy. Women accede to dominance hierarchies because of "the one terrible threat that never goes away"[43]—the need of females to have protection from killer males, who will injure or kill not only females but also the children that females guard. The battering that women suffer from the males they live with is the price paid for such protection, and occurs "in species where females have few allies, or where males have bonds with each other."[44] Indeed, among humans, sex differences trump the blood ties associated with natural selection for inclusive fitness. As anthropologist Barbara D. Miller notes,

> Human gender hierarchies are one of the most persistent, pervasive, and pernicious forms of inequality in the world. Gender is used as the basis for systems of discrimination which can, even within the same household, provide that those designated "male" receive more food and live longer, while those designated "female" receive less food to the point that their survival is drastically impaired.[45]

The sex with physical power also dominates political power, so that when law developed in human societies, men created legal systems that, generally speaking, favored male reproductive success and interests—with adultery as a crime for women but not for men; with female infanticide, male-on-female domestic violence, and marital rape not recognized as crimes; with polygyny legal but polyandry proscribed; with divorce easy for men and almost impossible for women.

FEMALE ADAPTIVE CHOICES MAY HELP PERPETUATE VIOLENT PATRIARCHY The development of male dominance hierarchies may also alter female evolution, and females apparently begin to make adaptive choices that serve to perpetuate this system. Primary among these female choices that entrench violent patriarchy are a general preference for the most dominant men

certain behavioral proclivities induced by the "strange path" our ancestors took; Wrangham and Peterson argue:

Men have a vastly long history of violence [which] implies that they have been temperamentally shaped to use violence effectively, and that they will therefore find it hard to stop. It is startling, perhaps, to recognize the absurdity of the system: one that works to benefit our genes rather than our conscious selves, and that inadvertently jeopardizes the fate of all our descendants.[50]

In other words, the foreign policy of human groups, including modern states, is more dangerous because of the human male evolutionary legacy:

Unfortunately, there appears something special about foreign policy in the hands of males. Among humans and chimpanzees at least, male coalitionary groups often go beyond defense [typical of monkey matriarchies] to include unprovoked aggression, which suggests that our own intercommunity conflicts might be less terrible if they were conducted on behalf of women's rather than men's interests. Primate communities organized around male interests naturally tend to follow male strategies and, thanks to sexual selection, tend to seek power with an almost unbounded enthusiasm.[51]

Thayer concurs, noting that "war evolved in humans because it is an effective way to gain and defend resources."[52] Moreover, because the evolutionary environment produced egoism, domination, and the in-group/out-group distinction, "these specific traits are sufficient to explain why state leaders will maximize their power over others and their environment, even if they must hurt others or risk injury to themselves."[53] Indeed, the title of Thayer's book speaks to the point: *Darwin and International Relations*. He finds ultimate cause for such observable modern state-level phenomena as offensive realism and ethnic conflict in natural selection.[54] Potts and Hayden note, "[M]ale Homo sapiens . . . have an inherited predisposition to team up with kin—or *perceived kin*—and try to kill their neighbors" (emphasis added).[55] It is important to note, then, that nationalist identity can substitute for biological kin ties in the perverse logic of male aggression.

Might there be selection within certain types of states for such "evolutionary" leaders? Political scientist Stephen Rosen believes so, and postulates

oping strong female alliances—male dominance is not order-wide among primates.

Second, cultural selection modifies natural selection through engineering of social structures and moral sanctions. Examples include how socially imposed monogamy, posited as leading to the depersonalization of power through democracy and capitalism, helped to open the way for improved status for women.[59] Another example is offered by the historian Mary Hartman, whose research has demonstrated that when northwestern Europe began in the twelfth century to break traditions of patrilocality and the marriage of pubescent girls to grooms ten years older, this unprecedented one-two punch to the traditional male dominance hierarchy that structured society created equally unprecedented changes in societal attitudes about many things, including governance. Indeed, Hartman believes that it was the more egalitarian marriages of northwestern Europe that set the stage for the rise of sustainable democracy (and capitalism) in human society.

Long before the contingent nature of the marital contract was recognized in law, marriages were conducted in northwestern Europe as joint enterprises by the two adult members, each of whom had recognized and reciprocal duties and obligations. In circumstances that required both members of an alliance to work and postpone marriage until there was a sufficient economic base to establish a household, individual self-reliance was a requirement long before individualism itself became an abstract social and political ideal. A sense of equality of rights was further promoted by such arrangements long before notions of egalitarianism became the popular coin of political movements. These later marriages, forged now through consent by the adult principals, offered themselves as implicit models to the sensibilities of political and religious reformers grappling with questions of authority. Experience in families, which were miniature contract societies unique to northwestern Europe, offers a plausible explanation for popular receptivity to the suggestion that the state itself rests upon a prior and breakable contract with all its members. And if this is so, the influence of family organization on the ways people were coming to conceive and shape the world at large can hardly be exaggerated. The lingering mystery about the origins of a movement of equal rights and individual freedom can be explained. Contrary to notions that these were imported items, it appears that they, along with charity, began at home.[60]

that emphasize an adaptive genetic basis, would not include the interacting influences of male privilege, social power, and the status of women—social and cultural dimensions of rape.[66] Instead of conceptualizing rape within a singular theoretical framework, rape and all violence against women should be understood within a contextual developmental model that integrates factors across several levels of analysis, examining not only individual differences but individual behavior in the context of intergenerational patterns and traditions as well as social-political objectives, including war.[67] Certain intrapersonal variables predict violence against women, but only in specific historical and sociocultural environments. Embedded in networks of families, peers, and work are characteristics of the personal relationships in which individuals commit microaggressive acts.

THE ENVIRONMENT IS CRITICALLY INVOLVED IN SHAPING MALE VIOLENCE AGAINST WOMEN Archer's meta-analytic review of sex differences in aggression between heterosexual partners in Western societies found that women were slightly more likely than men to have used physical aggression and to have used it more frequently.[68] Men were more likely to inflict injury because of their greater physical strength. However, these findings are based on studies of modern Western societies where men are taught that they should use restraint when it comes to physical aggression toward women. The results would likely not be replicated in countries with substantially different cultures, where violence against women is condoned, where patriarchal beliefs that men are responsible for controlling their wives' behavior are predominant, or where traditions inhibiting men from hitting women are absent. John Archer reports that ethnographic records further show that aggression by men toward women is more common where male alliances are strong and where men have power over resources. In addition, Archer's comprehensive meta-analyses of sex differences in aggression from real-world studies found that men used more dangerous acts of physical aggression. These sex differences were consistent across those nations for which there was evidence.[69]

Social role theorists, such as Alice Eagly and Wendy Wood, argue, however, that sex differences in human behavior do not lie mainly in evolved dispositions, but in the differing placement of women and men in the social structure.[70] Both positions focus on a functional analysis of behavior that emphasizes adjustment to environmental conditions. Here social role theory purports that sex differences emerge primarily from physical sex differences in conjunction with influences of the social constraints under which men

a child's engaging in antisocial behavior.[77] Significant increases in antisocial behaviors occur when an adopted child has both a genetic factor and an adverse environmental factor present. Again, the number of antisocial behaviors attributable to the presence of both genetic and environmental factors is far greater than the predicted increase from either factor acting alone.[78] Kenneth Dodge and Michelle Sherrill review findings that provide robust support for a person-environment interaction effect and argue that because maltreatment of children also alters biological processes in neural brain development, biology and the environment do not merely interact but transact across development.[79]

After further analyses, Raine concludes that environmental influences may even alter gene expression to trigger the cascade of events that translate genes into antisocial behavior.[80] Furthermore, according to Steve Cole, the relationship between genes and social behavior has historically been construed as a one-way street, with genes in control.[81] Recent analyses have challenged this view by discovering broad alterations in the expression of human genes as a function of differing socio-environmental conditions. Thus it appears that "the experience of environment not only 'gets inside the body' but 'stays there' in a concrete molecular way that propagates through multiple gene-transcriptional responses, physiologic systems, and time epochs."[82] Frances Champagne and Rahia Mashoodh also argue that there is evidence of the inheritance of environmentally induced effects, reflected in the findings of the new field of epigenetics, which provides further support for the notion that the transmission of traits across generations is not limited to the inheritance of DNA.[83]

These findings underscore the importance of the environment, not only because it is a critical determinant of whether violence against women will occur, but also because it is involved in perpetuating this type of violence over generations. Thus, an analysis of the social learning processes contributing to such gender-based violence as infanticide and sex trafficking provides a more complete explanation of how these heinous practices have come about, as well as a blueprint for designing strategies that will decrease them.

INDIVIDUALS ARE ACTUALLY TRAINED TO BE VIOLENT AGAINST WOMEN Although many studies have concluded that among preschool-age children, boys are more physically aggressive than girls,[84] when the stimulus of gender is removed[85] there is no difference between the amount of aggression boys display against girls and the amount girls display against boys.[86] This

Violence and coercion must "work" for these behaviors to be perpetuated or, in the parlance of evolutionary theory, "selected for." The reactions of parents, siblings, and peers train children to select actions that work and to ignore those that do not, to repeat responses that are functional and drop responses that are nonfunctional. For example, Thayer notes, "[c]ulture allows warfare to be either suppressed or exacerbated. . . . It is difficult to overstate the significance of educational systems, popular culture, and the media, among many [proximate] causal mechanisms."[95] It is the environment that determines the nature of the fittest response.[96] Here we glimpse the proximate causes of cultural selection in the very act.

The simple fact is that behavior is not regularly engaged in unless it is serving some purpose important to the individual. Furthermore, as the magnitude of the reinforcement increases, the acquisition of the behavior is faster, the rate of responding is higher, and resistance to extinction is greater. Individuals would not commit violent acts against women unless such violence benefited the perpetrators in some way. Sometimes the consequences solve a problem,[97] or alleviate an adversity.[98] The selling of a child bride, for example, might protect the family from the possibility of dishonor that would come should the child become promiscuous as a teenager, or perhaps such a transaction would provide income for a starving family. Many wife batterers have reported that they are violent in order to control their partners and assert themselves as powerful and in charge.[99] Child molesters, rapists, and serial sexual killers consistently reveal erotically charged violence, with sexual satisfaction obtained either overtly or symbolically.[100] Other reported rewards for violating women include the use of rape as revenge, with women viewed as collectively liable for the perpetrators' problems, or as a particularly exciting form of impersonal sex, in which women are viewed as sexual commodities to be used rather than as human beings with rights and feelings.[101]

While peers play a key role in reinforcing violent behavior, often the reinforcement comes directly from the victim in the form of submission, crying, or pain.[102] Under these circumstances, violence against women is immediately reinforced. Sexual coercion and marital rape are almost always related to fulfilling the emotional or physical needs of men.[103] Such violence provides immediate and intense gratification. Sex, itself, is a powerful reinforcer that fulfills a basic physical need for survival of the species. Furthermore, the selfish satisfaction inherent in this type of male domination is often justified by cultural and religious traditions that are themselves results of social diffusion, and that in turn offer additional social rewards for the perpetrator's aggression.

boys to have access to more food, the message is immediately sent that female children are of less value than male children and that little girls should not be given the same opportunities that are given to little boys. The discriminatory act against girls is followed by boys obtaining more food, which serves as a powerful reinforcer in any situation but particularly where food is scarce. As time goes on, boys are continually inundated with examples of adults' demonstrating their lack of value for female life and female work, with each example followed by reinforcing advantages given to boys and men. These adult models that children first observe imposing such gender inequities are usually their parents or other caregivers of the children. As such, these adults are the sources of affection and protection for their children and therefore have enormous influence on them.

In homes where interparental violence occurs, children who witness such violence are susceptible to adopting the aggressive behavior patterns they observe.[107] Children who witness violence between their parents are more likely to be violent with their peers and with their partners in future relationships; this is particularly true for males.[108] Those children found to be most violent are sons of abusers, following in their fathers' footsteps by becoming violent in the same types of conflicts that trigger their fathers' violence.[109] Sons' imitation of their fathers' aggression toward their mothers may be the first step in perpetuating patterns of violence against women across generations.

MALE AFFILIATION LEADS MEN TO PREFER MALE COMPANY AND TO ASSOCIATE WITH OTHER MEN In concert with findings of evolutionary biology concerning male coalitions, studies of children have repeatedly found evidence that boys prefer to play with boys.[110] Bonnie Ballif-Spanvill and her coauthors found that when three-year-old boys play with other three-year-old boys, the amount of prosocial behavior between them significantly increases.[111] Findings show that as early as six years of age, males form more durable bonds than females do with unrelated same-sex individuals.[112] This male camaraderie may be not only the foundation for same-gender preferences observed in children at play, but also the dynamics observed in everyday anecdotal activities of athletic teams and male-only clubs.

Clear evidence has demonstrated that when compared to females, males exhibit a higher threshold of tolerance for genetically unrelated same-sex individuals.[113] Across diverse cultures, males form larger, more inclusive, and more interconnected networks than females and exhibit greater cooperation among unrelated males. The authors conclude that their studies provide evidence that compared with females, males should be able to cooperate with

about women, the associations were stronger.[124] Groups of men who accept violence in relationships, believe that women deserve violence, and think that it is men's place to be dominant are much more likely to be violent against women.

THE MALE IN-GROUP VIEWS FEMALES AS AN INFERIOR OUT-GROUP

Although there is overwhelming evidence that young children favor their in-group, they do not engage in out-group derogation. When it does occur, it appears that children are simply reproducing attitudes held by adult members of particular national contexts.[125] Evidence does exist that men respond more strongly than women to intergroup threats.[126] When conflicts become more intense or circumstances more dire, adult in-group members display more extreme misperceptions and distorted judgments of the out-group. According to Ervin Staub, persistent difficulties of life also disrupt the relationships among members of the group because people focus on their own needs and compete with others for resources.[127] Threats and frustrations give rise to hostility, but the appropriate targets of this hostility usually cannot be identified or are too powerful to be reached; hence the hostility is displaced and directed toward substitute targets, often women who are already devalued and whose suffering is viewed as deserved. Goldstein believes that men adhere more strongly than women do to an in-group versus an out-group psychology and are, therefore, inherently more hostile toward outsiders, more able to demonize and dehumanize an enemy, and hence more willing to be violent and even kill.[128]

Particular attention should be paid to Donelson Forsyth's discussion of groups and power.[129] He says that individuals vary in their desire for power, but power holders who are very secure in their position may overstep the bounds of their authority and become preoccupied with gaining more. Further evidence has been found that shows that higher-power individuals have less compassion in response to another person's suffering.[130] In addition, violence among the powerful has been found to be a result of a threatened ego.[131] In these studies, individuals with power became aggressive when they felt incompetent in the domain of their power. Here the behavior of the powerful is not unlike the behavior of men involved in domestic violence who compensate for their lack of marital power with physical aggression.[132]

WHERE MALE GROUPS CONDONE VIOLENCE AGAINST WOMEN, THEY PERCEIVE WOMEN AS ENEMIES AND THUS JUSTIFY VIOLENCE AGAINST THEM In terms of deviant behavior and partner violence,

LACK OF FEMALE AFFILIATION RESULTS IN WOMEN'S ALLEGIANCE TO MALE AUTHORITIES Female children or adults do not appear to have as positive same-sex compatibility, comparable to that found among males. Even at three months of age, both sexes preferred to attend to the male peers.[141] These findings, coupled with the fact that in most societies, women are structurally organized in patrilocal families under the direction of men, could explain why even when women associate with other women, their allegiance is primarily to the male heads of their households. As previously discussed, this may also be a tragic by-product of human evolution as it pertains to female choice.

SOCIAL ENGINEERING OF THESE PROXIMATE CAUSES CAN COUNTERACT VIOLENCE AGAINST WOMEN The special contribution of psychology to the women and peace thesis is the identification of the discrete proximate causes that can be manipulated to counteract and even undermine violent patriarchy. Very young boys are not demonstrably prone to aggression against girls; it takes active modeling, reinforcement, and rewarding of gendered violence to make it appear functional to boys. If it is not modeled, if it is not reinforced, if it is actively punished, its incidence can be severely limited. These are proximate causes that humans can consciously control. If gendered microaggression and violence can be undermined at its taproot—domestic violence within the home—the effects, as we have shown with violent patriarchy, should cascade outward to affect many social phenomena, including state security and behavior. Furthermore, if institutions can be created that depersonalize political power, thus severing its connection to power within a male dominance hierarchy, then legal systems and political institutions that allow females to live free of violence from males, and therefore free to form countervailing female alliances to prevent male violence and dominance, will also have a profound effect on state security and behavior. To the extent that the security of women is a societal priority, the security and peacefulness of the state will be significantly enhanced. State security rests, in the first place, on the security of women.

POLITICAL SOCIOLOGY AND SOCIAL DIFFUSION

From the view of evolutionary theorists that the primal character of violent patriarchy ensures that it becomes a template for broad classes of social behavior that concern social difference, and from the contributions of social psychologists' and political sociologists' analyses of subtle but strong environmental

lower levels of gender inequality hinder the ability of societies to mobilize for aggression through the denigration of women.[147]

PERVASIVE STRUCTURAL VIOLENCE AND SYSTEMATIC EXPLOITATION DESCRIBE THE MEANS BY WHICH GENDER INEQUALITY IS TYPICALLY MAINTAINED WITHIN A SOCIETY Johan Galtung, a political scientist specializing in political sociology, offers two concepts that help explain how a generalized ideological justification for violence is formed and diffuses throughout society: structural violence and cultural violence.[148] Galtung's conceptualization of structural violence paints a picture of pervasive and systematic exploitation that makes open violence in the public sphere unnecessary: "The amateur who wants to dominate uses guns, the professional uses social structure."[149] According to Galtung, structural violence has at least four manifestations: exploitation based on a division of labor wherein benefits are asymmetrically distributed; control by the exploiters over the consciousness of the exploited, resulting in the acquiescence of the oppressed; fragmentation, meaning that the exploited are separated from each other; and marginalization, with the exploiters as a privileged class who have their own rules and form of interaction.[150]

The concordance between this list and the means by which gender inequality is typically maintained in human societies is clear. Gender roles lead to highly differential possibilities for personal security, development, and prosperity, even in today's world. An example of this kind of exploitation occurs when women "naturally" receive less pay than men for equal work, or when domestic violence is considered "normal." The second component, manipulation of consciousness to ensure acquiescence, is maintained through socialization, gender stereotyping, and a constant threat of domestic violence—all of which insidiously identify women as inferior. The perpetrators of female infanticide, for example, are virtually all female. The third component, fragmentation, is easily effected from women's circumstances of patrilocality, economic prostration, and greater family responsibilities (and in some cases, a physical purdah may be used), thus minimizing social access that could otherwise be used to build networks with other women. And finally, marginalization serves to clearly distinguish men and women, with no doubt as to the relative status of each sex.

STRUCTURAL VIOLENCE IS BASED ON CULTURAL VIOLENCE—THAT IS, OPEN OR IMPLICIT VIOLENCE IN PRIVATE SPHERES Galtung posits that structural violence arises from cultural violence—the day-to-day use of

4

THE HEART OF THE MATTER

The Security of Women and the Security of States

What are the roots of conflict and insecurity for states? Attention turns to differences in state attributes when the international system is relatively stable. Some scholars argue that civilizational differences, defined by ethnicity, language, and religion, are an underlying catalyst for conflict and insecurity.[1] Others have spoken of the importance of differentiating between democratic and nondemocratic regime types in explaining conflict in the modern international system.[2] Still others assert that poverty, exacerbated by resource scarcity in a context of unequal access, is at the heart of conflict and insecurity at both micro levels and macro levels of analysis.[3]

In this chapter, we argue that there is another fundamental and powerful explanatory factor that must be considered when examining issues of state security and conflict: the treatment of females within society. At first glance, this argument seems hardly intuitive. How could the treatment of women possibly be linked to matters of high politics, such as war and national security? The two realms seem not to inhabit the same conceptual space. Yet in 2006, Secretary-General of the United Nations Kofi Annan opined, "The world is starting to grasp that there is no policy more effective in promoting development, health, and education than the empowerment of women and girls. And I would venture that no policy is more important in preventing conflict, or in achieving reconciliation after a conflict has ended."[4] It is possible that views such as Annan's are just a nod to political correctness, which can be ignored without consequence by security scholars and policymakers. Yet it is also possible that security scholars are missing something important by overlooking the situation of women in the study of security. In this chapter, we wish to

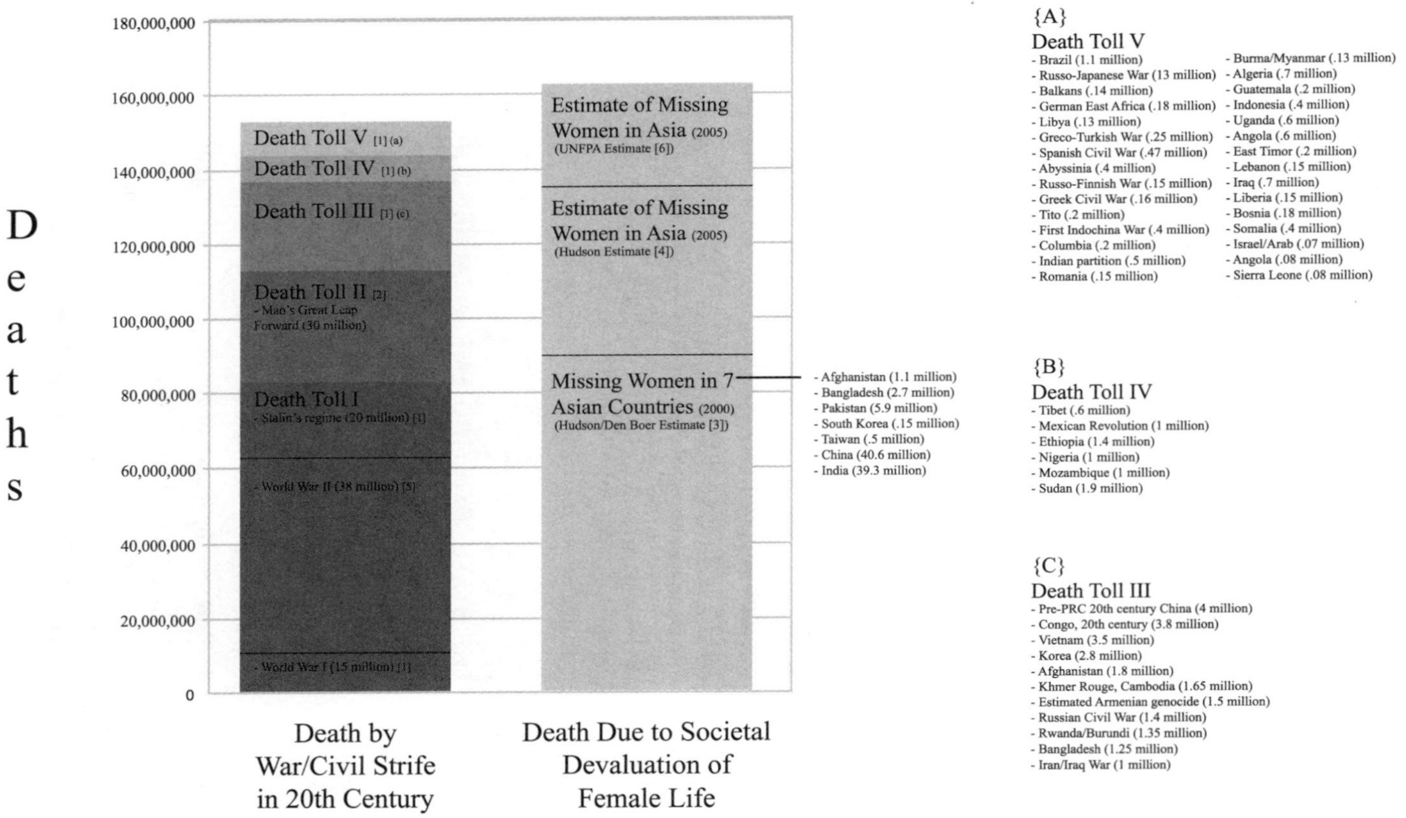

Death Due to Societal Devaluation of Female Life

Death by War/Civil Strife in 20th Century

Deaths

180,000,000
160,000,000
140,000,000
120,000,000
100,000,000
80,000,000
60,000,000
40,000,000
20,000,000
0

Death Toll V [1](a)
Death Toll IV [1](b)
Death Toll III [1](c)
Death Toll II [2] - Mao's Great Leap Forward (30 million)
Death Toll I - Stalin's regime (20 million) [1]
World War II (38 million) [5]
World War I (15 million) [1]

Estimate of Missing Women in Asia (2005) (UNFPA Estimate [6])
Estimate of Missing Women in Asia (2005) (Hudson Estimate [4])
Missing Women in 7 Asian Countries (2000) (Hudson/Den Boer Estimate [3])
- Afghanistan (1.1 million)
- Bangladesh (2.7 million)
- Pakistan (5.9 million)
- South Korea (.15 million)
- Taiwan (.5 million)
- China (40.6 million)
- India (39.3 million)

{A}
Death Toll V
- Brazil (1.1 million)
- Russo-Japanese War (13 million)
- Balkans (.14 million)
- German East Africa (.18 million)
- Libya (.13 million)
- Greco-Turkish War (25 million)
- Spanish Civil War (47 million)
- Abyssinia (.4 million)
- Russo-Finnish War (.15 million)
- Greek Civil War (.16 million)
- Tito (2 million)
- Columbia (.2 million)
- Indian partition (.5 million)
- Romania (.15 million)
- Burma/Myanmar (.13 million)
- Algeria (.7 million)
- Guatemala (.2 million)
- Indonesia (.4 million)
- Uganda (.6 million)
- Angola (.6 million)
- East Timor (.2 million)
- Lebanon (.15 million)
- Iraq (.7 million)
- Liberia (.15 million)
- Bosnia (.18 million)
- Somalia (.4 million)
- Israel/Arab (.07 million)
- Angola (.08 million)
- Sierra Leone (.08 million)

{B}
Death Toll IV
- Tibet (.6 million)
- Mexican Revolution (1 million)
- Ethiopia (1.4 million)
- Nigeria (1 million)
- Mozambique (1 million)
- Sudan (1.9 million)

{C}
Death Toll III
- Pre-PRC 20th century China (4 million)
- Congo, 20th century (3.8 million)
- Vietnam (3.5 million)
- Korea (2.8 million)
- Afghanistan (1.8 million)
- Khmer Rouge, Cambodia (1.65 million)
- Estimated Armenian genocide (1.5 million)
- Russian Civil War (1.4 million)
- Rwanda/Burundi (1.35 million)
- Bangladesh (1.25 million)
- Iran/Iraq War (1 million)

FIGURE 4.1 Comparison of Conflict Deaths in the Twentieth Century and Deaths Resulting from Devaluation of Female Life at the Turn of the Twenty-first Century

child survival/mortality and malnutrition, are also significantly correlated to female status and education.[15]

Besides the linkages between the situation and status of women, on the one hand, and economic and health variables on the other, we are now beginning to see research on political variables also. We have already noted the negative correlation between indices of corruption and indices of women's social and economic rights.[16] Women's rights thus offer an added economic benefit: because decreases in political corruption increase investment and growth, gender equity additionally promotes economic growth.[17] Furthermore, the priorities and perspectives of the government may change as women become more visible and audible within its ranks. Remember the research that we surveyed in chapter 2: studies show that the more women in government, the greater the attention given to social welfare, legal protection, and transparency in government and business. In one survey, 80 percent of respondents said that women's participation restores trust in government.[18] All in all, then, the world is beginning to recognize that the status of women often substantially influences important aspects of the states in which they live. This recognition, in turn, has led to innovative policy initiatives to capitalize on these insights.[19]

Despite this impressive array of empirical findings, when one turns to questions of women and national security defined in a more traditional sense, questions still remain. Although there are theoretical reasons for believing that the security and behavior of a state is linked to the situation and security of its women, does the evidence support this proposition? And what is the form of that linkage? These questions have not been as exhaustively researched as has the linkage between the situation of women and the prosperity/health of nations.

There are two primary strands of inquiry that have brought this linkage into sharper focus: academic theory and policy exposition. A strong foundation in the rich theoretical literature of feminist security studies emphasizes the relationship between women's status and international relations, and we urge our readers to begin an enlightening journey of discovery by delving into these works.[20] In addition to academic endeavors, noteworthy is the formal articulation of the need to include women in peace negotiations as codified in the 2000 UN Security Council Resolution 1325, the 2008 recognition in UN Security Council Resolution 1820 of the need to punish those who commit rape in conflict, a broader IGO/NGO advocacy program called Women,

pression, including authoritarianism, in Islamic nation-states. Treatment of women, then, may affect societal propensity to adopt a particular governance system, such as authoritarianism or democracy.

Another primary question of interest is how the treatment of women at the domestic level has an impact on state behavior internationally. This question is important to show the linkage between gender and security because it shows those with decision-making power that the treatment of women has far-reaching consequences well beyond that of social justice. The international system may be more or less secure depending upon the situation of women within its units. A body of conventional empirical work spearheaded by Mary Caprioli links measures of domestic gender inequality to state-level variables concerning conflict and security, with statistically significant results. Caprioli uses four measures of gender equality—political equality (percentage of women in parliament and number of years of suffrage), economic equality (percentage of women in the labor force), and social equality (fertility rate)—to show that states with higher levels of social, economic, and political gender equality are less likely to rely on military force to settle international disputes.[27] In other words, Caprioli found that higher levels of gender equality make a state less likely to threaten, display, or use force, or go to war once involved in an interstate dispute. Caprioli argues that foreign policy aimed at creating peace should focus on improving the status of women.

Caprioli and Mark Boyer examine the impact of gender equality on a state's behavior during international crises, which is a situation in which there is a high probability of violence. They wanted to find out whether gender equality has an impact on state behavior when violence is highly likely. They show that states exhibiting high levels of gender equality measured by the percentage of women in parliament also exhibit lower levels of violence in international crises and disputes.[28] Examining aggregate data over a fifty-year period (1954–1994), they found a statistically significant relationship between level of violence in crisis and the percentage of female leaders. In general, states with higher levels of political gender equality are less likely to have minor clashes, serious clashes, or war in the high-stakes environment of international crisis. As did Caprioli's inquiry, the research by Caprioli and Boyer finds that gender equality has an effect on a state's foreign policy behavior in terms of decreasing violence during international crises.

Thus far, we have examined the literature showing that gender equality matters when states are involved in interstate disputes and when they are involved in international crises. This literature does not examine the process

disputes, to use violence during militarized disputes, to use force first during militarized disputes, to increase the severity of violence during international crises, and to become involved in civil conflicts. The status of women, it seems, is a taproot of international security.

Furthermore, the relative absence of women's perspectives and voices in the society's decision-making councils may also have a negative effect on prospects for peace. Rose McDermott and Jonathan Cowden examine sex differences in aggression with the context of a simulated crisis game.[34] In these experiments, all-female pairs proved significantly less likely than all-male pairs to spend money on weapons procurement or to go to war in the face of a crisis. In further research, McDermott and her coauthors found that in simulation, males are more likely to display overconfidence prior to gaming, and are more likely to use unprovoked violence as a tactic.[35] These types of simulations, despite their constraints, permit the inclusion of sex-based psychological variables in theories concerning the micro processes by which gender differences might affect resulting state security processes and outcomes.[36]

Indeed, perhaps Samuel Huntington's reflections on the clash of civilizations between nations would be better viewed as a clash between gender civilizations, with treatment of women being an important marker of civilizational divide.[37] Ronald Inglehart and Pippa Norris, though not researching nation-state behavior per se, examined psychological attitudes toward women across "civilizations" defined more traditionally in terms of religion or ethnicity. They found that contrary to popular impression, beliefs about democracy and other political values are not very different between, say, Islamic and Christian cultures. Beliefs about gender equality, however, differ markedly, which they take to be evidence that conceptualization of culture, or the nation-state, or civilization must be redefined to include a gender component. Furthermore, they find strong associations between psychological attitudes about women and indicators such as the percentage of women elected to the national legislature.[38]

These findings are encouraging: using conventional methodologies, we can glimpse aspects of the relationship we would expect to find between the security of women and the security of states. We have subjected the women-and-peace thesis to further empirical testing, specifically including a examination of levels of violence against women as a predictor of state peacefulness. After surveying our sources of information, we will present our research findings to date.

der Empowerment Measure (GEM) and Gender Development Index (GDI). These oft-used indices, though pioneering, still leave much to be desired in light of the research agenda we wish to pursue, because they rely on less than half a dozen of the most often used statistics, primarily those cited above, and they omit measures of violence against women. The newly announced GII (Gender Inequality Index), is set to replace both GDI and GEM, but still shares some of its predecessors' problems. In addition to GEM and GDI, the CIRI Human Rights Dataset has also developed three indices of women's rights.[40] These include four-point indices of women's political rights, women's economic rights, and women's social rights, and CIRI is to be commended for its attempt to include gender-sensitive indicators in its dataset. At the same time, the CIRI index seeks to capture the stance taken by the government, not the actual situation of women in the country.

The Gender Gap Index (GGI) of the World Economic Forum (WEF) is the most ambitious project to date in efforts to more fully capture the situation of women. The WEF has developed eight scales. The coding for four of the scales is obscure (paternal versus maternal authority, polygamy, female genital mutilation, and the existence of laws punishing violence against women). The coding for the other four scales, however—economic participation and opportunity (five statistics), educational attainment (four statistics), political empowerment (three statistics), and health and survival (two statistics)—contains the usual half dozen statistics, as cited above, plus variants; for example, educational attainment looks at gaps not only in female-to-male literacy but also in enrollment figures at the primary, secondary, and tertiary levels. This is an impressive achievement, but we cannot help but notice that once again important variables concerning the status of women—for example, rates of violence against women—are not compiled. All of the scales evidence a persistent reliance on easily quantified information, to the exclusion of qualitative information that could provide a more nuanced view of the situation of women. The United Nations Economic Commission on Africa's AGDI (African Gender and Development Index) comes much closer to our ideal of multifactorial, qualitative-plus-quantitative measures used as the foundation for a richer scaling of the cross-national status of women, but it was scaled for only twelve sub-Saharan African nations.[41]

Researchers seeking to study the impact of gender inequality on state security and behavior are thus faced with a serious challenge. There are approximately six to ten variables concerning women that are easily quantified and that form the basis for most analysis of the situation of women in the

state-level phenomena related to security. Furthermore, the degree of association should meet or exceed that of established alternative hypotheses.

What state-level phenomena related to security might be related to the security of women? The literature has already confirmed a linkage to state-level variables indicating the relative health and prosperity of nations. Though these are certainly related to the concept of security, here we wish to use variables that are traditionally associated with "national security." These would include data on whether the state was involved in intrastate or interstate conflict, whether the state demonstrated an aggressive foreign policy, whether the state used force first in an interstate dispute, whether the state was compliant with international norms as set down in United Nations treaties and covenants, whether the nation had friendly or unfriendly relations with its neighbors and other members of the international system, and so forth.

Although this discussion suggests many possible indicators of state security, in this empirical analysis we focus primarily on three measures as dependent variables. First, we examine a general measure of state peacefulness (the Global Peace Index, or GPI). The GPI score incorporates twenty-four indicators, including external conflicts, civil conflicts, and military expenditures. Second, we investigate a general measure of the degree of behavioral deviancy of the state in light of international norms (the States of Concern to the International Community, or SOCIC scale). This scale, which overlaps in conceptualization with the GPI, also includes information, absent in the GPI, on whether the state has violated certain security-related international treaties and covenants, such as the Nuclear Non-Proliferation Treaty, or the Convention Against Torture. Third, we analyze one of the GPI subcomponent indicators, Neighbouring Countries Relations (RN). Dominance hierarchies rooted in the domination of one sex by the other should manifest their dysfunctionality in relations with neighboring countries, even if they do not possess the capabilities to project dominance in a global sense.

In this exploratory empirical analysis, we examine the following hypotheses that probe the linkage between the security of women and the security of states:

THE PHYSICAL SECURITY OF WOMEN H1. Higher levels of women's physical security will exhibit significant and positive statistical association with the Global Peace Index, the States of Concern to the International Community Scale, and the Relations with Neighbors subcomponent of GPI.

H2. As measured by polytomous logistic regression pseudo-R-squared values in both bivariate and multivariate analysis,[44] measures of the physical

feminist security studies believe that conventional notions of causality do not apply when phenomena are co-constitutive and that violence against women and state violence may well be co-constitutive. In this view, if scholars must confine themselves to an arbitrary temporal separation to show causality, co-constitutive phenomena will defy the logic of conventional empirical investigation—perhaps ruling out the very notion of a gendered analysis.[46]

We do aspire one day to conventionally ascertain causality through temporal extension of the Physical Security of Women (PSOW) Scale, but here we must content ourselves with assessing the significance of association in the context of what we think are strong theoretical reasons to believe that dominance hierarchies rooted in evolutionary human male reproductive strategies do create templates of violence that diffuse through society widely, affecting even state behavior in relation to internal and external entities. In a sense, what we are probing for is whether the degree of mitigation of the primal templates of violent patriarchy (measured as variation in the prevalence and level of violence against women) is reflected in mitigation of state insecurity and violence. The greater the mitigation of the first, the greater we should find the mitigation of the second to be. This stance does not rule out the possibility that state insecurity and violence in turn exaggerate the insecurity of women.

OPERATIONALIZATIONS

To test the hypotheses listed above, each variable must be operationalized. Information on all variables utilized, with their associated operationalizations, is available in appendix A. Briefly, the variables used in the analysis include PSOW (Physical Security of Women; WomanStats), PSOWSP (Physical Security of Women including Son Preference, WomanStats), PSOWMMR (Physical Security of Women Minus Marital Rape; WomanStats), GPI (Global Peace Index; Economist Intelligence Unit; used as a dependent variable); SOCIC (States of Concern to the International Community, Carl Brinton; used as a dependent variable), RN (Neighboring Countries Relations (Economist Intelligence Unit; used as a dependent variable), Level of Organized Intrastate Conflict (Economist Intelligence Unit; used as a dependent variable), Level of Democracy (Freedom House; used as a control variable), Level of Wealth (GDP per capita quintile; CIA World Factbook; used as a control variable), Prevalence of Islamic Civilization (Stearmer and Emmett; used as a control variable), IFL (Inequity in Family Law/Practice; WomanStats), Prevalence of

These results indicate that the prevalence of Islamic culture is not, comparatively speaking, an important predictor of the level of peacefulness of the state, or of the degree to which a state is of concern to the international community, or of the quality of relations between the state and its neighbors. The pseudo-R-squared values for level of democracy, wealth, and the physical security of women are all much higher than those for Islamic culture, and in multivariate analysis this variable is not a significant discriminator (see table B.2 in appendix B for full multivariate results).

In comparing bivariate regression results for the three alternative independent variables, the highest pseudo-R-squareds are obtained for the measure of the physical security of women. In three of the four possible comparisons (level of democracy/physical security of women in reference to GPI; level of wealth/physical security of women in reference to SOCIC; and level of democracy/physical security of women in reference to RN), the physical security of women obviously outperforms the other explanatory variables. In the fourth possible comparison (level of democracy/physical security of women in reference to SOCIC), the pseudo-R-squareds are too close to represent a meaningful difference, though technically the pseudo-R-squared for the physical security of women measure is higher than that for level of democracy.

Multivariate regression is a critical next step, as it allows us to control for the alternative independent variables. Though space does not permit all three tables of multivariate results to be included, table B.3 in appendix B presents the multivariate regression of GPI on all four independent variables. In this analysis, the best significant discrimination is also obtained with the PSOW scale, as compared to the other three variables. Especially noteworthy in the multivariate analysis is that the discrimination afforded by PSOW obviously dwarfs that provided by level of democracy.

An additional test of the importance of the security of women for state peacefulness is to ask whether democracies, in particular, see their level of state peacefulness fall if their level of physical security of women worsens. The answer is yes. Tables B.4, B.5, and B.6 in appendix B examine the subset of full democracies (not "partially free" but fully "free" in the Freedom House terminology), dichotomized according to whether their PSOW score is low (o or 1) or higher (2, 3, or 4). (Note: Full cross-tabulation is provided only for GPI.) Does the first group enjoy greater state peacefulness (GPI), better compliance with international norms (SOCIC), and better relations

pendix B indicates that the association between IFL, on the one hand, and PSOW (MMR), on the other, is highly statistically significant using Pearson's r and Gamma, with significance measuring at $p < .0001$. Table B.12 in appendix B lists the Cox and Snell pseudo-R-squareds for *bivariate* regression of PSOW (MMR) on IFL, and also on the control variables, democracy, wealth, and prevalence of Islam. The results presented in table B.12 indicate that IFL clearly outperforms both democracy and prevalence of Islam in explaining the variance in PSOW. The desultory results of prevalence of Islam indicate that apparently there are several legal systems that encode inequitable evolutionary family law other than those found in Islam, and scholars would be remiss in focusing their attention solely on the inequities manifest in shari'a law. Furthermore, the Islamic nations are not uniform in their adherence to shari'a law, introducing a real spectrum of IFL scores within that group of nations.

Given that IFL is much more readily observable than physical security of women from a data collection standpoint, can we use IFL in the place of PSOW as a predictor of state peacefulness? Unsurprisingly, but importantly, 98 percent of the nations with nationally inequitable family law systems (IFL scale points 3 and 4) have high levels of societal violence against women (PSOW scale points 3 and 4), so this direction may be justified. Table B.13 presents bivariate Cox and Snell pseudo-R-squareds for each variable. These results indicate that IFL is a much better predictor of state peacefulness than either level of democracy or prevalence of Islamic civilization. In multivariate analysis (table B.14 in appendix B), we are able to see that level of wealth discriminates at only the highest scale point, not at any other scale point. Level of democracy provides no significant discrimination of state peacefulness at all, and neither does prevalence of Islamic civilization. However, the discrimination provided by IFL is impressive: by far the best predictor of state peacefulness in this analytic set is actually level of inequity in family law and practice.

DISCREPANCY BETWEEN STATE LAW AND SOCIETAL PRACTICE CONCERNING WOMEN If a state is indifferent about enforcing laws that protect the women in its society, is it also less likely to be compliant with international norms to which it has committed? We can examine this question by examining the association between the discrepancy between state law and societal practice concerning women variable on the one hand, and the SOCIC scale on the other. Table B.15 in appendix B shows that the results are very strong

WHAT IS SECURITY?

The results described above lead us to ask anew, What constitutes security? And how is security to be obtained? An account of security that does not include gender-based violence is an impoverished account of security. This is not so for reasons of political correctness; it is so on the basis of fairly robust, though preliminary, empirical findings. We find a strong and significant relationship between the physical security of women and the peacefulness of states. Furthermore, we believe there are sound theoretical reasons to expect this relationship to obtain. We assert that when evolutionary forces predisposing to violent patriarchy are not checked through the use of cultural selection and social learning to ameliorate gender inequality, dysfunctional templates of violence and control diffuse throughout society and are manifested in state security and behavior. Combining our present results with those of previous research efforts,[53] not only do we fail to falsify that theoretical assertion by using conventional aggregate statistical hypothesis-testing methodologies, but we find greater empirical warrant for that assertion than for several well-established alternative hypotheses.

We can now envision new research questions for security studies, which are possible to raise only if the linkage between the security of women and the security of states is taken seriously in that field. For example, terrorism is a topic that may profit from a gender analysis: Does polygamy lead to marriage market dislocations, which also heighten the allure of the terrorism among young adult males with no hope of eventually marrying?[54] Does the subjected status of women feed into the development of terrorist groups offering a promise of greater equality to women, such as we see in Sri Lanka and Nepal? Similarly, security demographics is a nascent subfield that, we argue, must incorporate gender lenses: for example, is enactment of son preference through female infanticide and sex-selective abortion a predisposing factor for state instability and bellicosity?[55] And what would Huntington's map look like if we re-drew it along the lines of differences in the security of women? Would we see a new type or definition of "civilization" by looking at that map, and would it give us greater leverage on questions of identity, conflict, and security than Huntington's original map? Are alliance patterns associated with membership in the same "gender civilization"? Is the recently noted ability of populations to increase their happiness set point over time linked to the improving security of women in those nations,[56] and what ramifications will that have for state behavior? In the subfield of foreign policy analysis,

a major, verging on suicidal, disadvantage for our species as a whole. . . . [T]o a very large extent . . . the natural tendencies of men are not consistent with the survival and well-being of their sexual partners, their children, and future generations to come.[57]

These questions will not subside in importance, but rather will grow in importance over time. We see in the current international system the rise to great power status of states in which the security of women is severely compromised. We cannot help but think of the rise of India and China, where almost a hundred million women are missing from the population as a result of sex-selective abortion, high suicide rates among young women, and other symptoms of a profound lack of security for women. We take this to mean that the true clash of civilizations in the future will not, in fact, be along the lines envisioned by Samuel Huntington but along the fault lines between civilizations that treat women as equal members of the human species and civilizations that cannot or will not do so. Furthermore, we expect to see much more prevalent conflict between and within nations of that second group.

FROM THEORY TO ACTION

In addition to these fresh new questions in the academic field of security studies, we must not overlook that women's status may actually be an integral element of any proposed solutions for international conflict. Though the treatment of women is written deeply in the culture of a society, it is amenable to change. Women have recently received the rights to vote and stand for office in countries where they have not had those rights before; UN Security Council Resolutions 1325 and 1820 have changed peacekeeping and conflict resolution practices on the ground; stricter enforcement of laws against sex-selective abortion is making a dent in abnormal birth sex ratios in some countries. There is no reason to shrug helplessly if we identify the insecurity of women as an important factor in state insecurity and conflict. To the contrary, the recognition that the security of women affects the security of states offers policymakers an inestimably valuable policy agenda in the quest for greater peace and stability in the international system.

In the view of Potts and Hayden, "Empowered women tend to counterbalance the most chaotic and violent aspects of men's predisposition for brutal territoriality and team aggression. . . . [I]n the human species, the empowerment of women and the possibility of peace and freedom . . . are united in

5

WINGS OF NATIONAL AND INTERNATIONAL RELATIONS, PART ONE

Effecting Positive Change Through Top-Down Approaches

THE ENORMITY OF THE THREE great inequities between men and women—the physical insecurity of women throughout the world, the gross inequity in family law in many parts of the world, and the relative absence of women in councils where the important decisions concerning human collectives are made—is daunting. Humankind has been likened to a bird with one strong wing (men) and one wounded wing (women), a bird that has never flown. How should human societies move to heal these wounds?

Contemplating this question, some think to pit top-down approaches against bottom-up approaches, asserting that one is more efficacious than the other. We view that discussion as a red herring: both approaches are necessary and must be used together in a pincer movement to effect lasting change. In this chapter, we will begin our examination of the dynamics of change by investigating the potential and the pitfalls of top-down policies to improve the security and situation of women.

WHY THE TOP MATTERS

The state possesses resources and capabilities that are simply not shared by other actors in society. Among these is the legitimate use of coercive violence. The power to detain, imprison, and even execute is capable of changing social norms, even those concerning women. The state can also coerce through nonviolent means, such as through its powers to impose fines or taxes upon activities that it wishes to discourage. Carrots are also available to the state, for it has the power to craft regulations, including tax and benefit codes, and

to write a series of success stories for USAID. All of them were in their 20s, 30s and 40s but looked to be in their 60s. Until very recently, none of them could work outside the home because they possessed no marketable skills, could neither read nor write and were unable to leave their homes for fear of being killed. Not one of them had less than five children and three of the seven had more than nine. A number of women mentioned that, prior to taking part in the programme—which focused on tailoring and basic literacy—their children used to weep at night from hunger.

As the reporter prepared to leave, the women fluttered around her like fragile moths, touching her sleeves and speaking all at once. "What are they saying?" asked the reporter to the young Pashto-speaking interpreter. "They are telling you to go back to your country and to ask your people not to abandon them," she replied.

"The women of Afghanistan don't want you to leave. They will quite literally die if the Taliban return," she said. Said the young interpreter as the reporter climbed back into the armoured SUV, "They will be killed or starved to death. Their [daughters] will be treated like dogs. They want you [to] return to your country and tell your leaders that the Coalition is their only hope." Importantly, every female foreign aid worker in Afghanistan I have met shares this view.[3]

In a recent question-and-answer period at one of our universities[4] (on his tour of sixty American universities), General David Petraeus was asked bluntly whether anyone thought to ask the women of Afghanistan how they felt about American hopes to incorporate "reformed" Taliban into governance structures as the Americans leave.

In an answer that carefully sidestepped the most important noun— "women"—the general assured the questioning student that only "moderate" Taliban would be eligible for such rehabilitation. Left unaddressed was the definition of "moderate," which clearly depends on where you sit: if you sit in a burqa, perhaps there is no such thing as a "moderate" Taliban. In fact, in talks with Hizb e-Islami, a Taliban group, one of its conditions for being "rehabilitated" is a return to its hard-line interpretation of shari'a law for all of Afghanistan.

Apparently, for the Americans, women (and by extension, as we have seen, prospects for peace) have taken a backseat to realpolitik and the exigencies of a Coalition exit strategy. Make no mistake: the decampment of the West will spell an end to efforts to bring equal rights to one-half of the Afghan population—and hope to a younger generation of moderates. Though

story on this was complex, one dissident asserted, "We Iranian men are late doing this. . . . If we did this when *rusari* [the headscarf] was forced on those among our sisters who did not wish to wear it 30 years ago, we would have perhaps not been here today."[8] This is a profound and poignant statement. Men who see women as beings who must be subjugated will themselves be forever subjugated. Men who see women as their equal and valued partners are the only men who have a true chance to win their freedom and enjoy peace. Indeed, as the empirical results of the previous chapter have shown, the most unstable societies are those that allow a high level of violence against women and control over women by men.

Furthermore, even from the point of view of the government, it is simply harder and more dangerous to rule a society where male-dominance hierarchies are not only condoned but actively promulgated. The alpha males of today will be the preferred targets of these hierarchies tomorrow. Who, then, wins from this system of "natural" hierarchy?

CEDAW

In concert with considering the power that states have to improve the lives of women in their society, it is important also to consider the broader international context. While there are many instruments that speak about human rights, such as the International Covenant on Civil and Political Rights, it has also been noted that unless a right is said to expressly belong to women, it may not in fact be assumed to do so. For this reason, in 1979 the Convention on the Elimination of All Forms of Discrimination Against Women was adopted by the UN General Assembly. CEDAW now has 186 state parties.[9] Indeed, the aforementioned Covenant on Civil and Political Rights has only 165 state parties. The International Covenant on Economic, Social, and Cultural Rights has only 160 state parties. In other words, more nations have become party to CEDAW than to the two oldest and most universal covenants on human rights.

CEDAW endeavors to be a bill of human rights for all women across the globe. It sets forth principles that embody equality, and it also defines what discrimination against women is. Nations acceding to the treaty agree to end discrimination against women in their laws and punish those who do not abide by these laws. Each state party is asked to present a report every four years that documents what actions the government is taking to implement CEDAW, and in what areas progress still needs to be made. These state

TABLE 5.1 Countries Posting Non-technical Reservations to CEDAW*

Algeria
Australia
Austria
Bahamas
Bahrain
Bangladesh
Brunei
Chile
DPRK (North Korea)
Egypt
France
India
Ireland
Israel
Jordan
Kuwait
Lebanon
Lesotho
Libya
Liechtenstein
Malaysia
Maldives
Malta
Mauritania
Mexico

(*continued*)

The Government of Finland recalls that by acceding to the Convention, a State commits itself to adopt the measures required for the elimination of discrimination, in all its forms and manifestations, against women.

A reservation which consists of a general reference to religious law and national law without specifying its contents, as the first part of the reservation made by Saudi Arabia, does not clearly define to other Parties to the Convention the extent to which the reserving State commits itself to the Convention and therefore creates serious doubts as to the commitment of the reserving State to fulfill its obligations under the Convention.

Furthermore, reservations are subject to the general principle of treaty interpretation according to which a party may not invoke the provisions of its domestic law as justification for a failure to perform its treaty obligations.

As the reservation to Paragraph 2 of Article 9 aims to exclude one of the fundamental obligations under the Convention, it is the view of the Government of Finland that the reservation is not compatible with the object and purpose of the Convention.

The Government of Finland also recalls Part VI, Article 28 of the Convention according to which reservations incompatible with the object and purpose of the Convention are not permitted.

The Government of Finland therefore objects to the above-mentioned reservations made by the Government of Saudi Arabia to the Convention.

This objection does not preclude the entry into force of the Convention between Saudi Arabia and Finland. The Convention will thus become operative between the two States without Saudi Arabia benefiting from the reservations.

5 March 2002

One of the most exciting recent developments in the area of CEDAW is the No Reservations Movement.[11] This movement, spearheaded by Muslim women, attempts to remove the reservations to CEDAW stipulated by many Islamic nations, particularly concerning articles 9–15, which address women's rights within the family, under what is variously termed "family law" or "personal status law." As anthropologist and noted Islamic feminist Ziba Mir-Hosseini said in a 2010 interview, "I think the issue of gender relations within the family—which is what personal status laws are all about—actually relates to the core of power in society at a broader level. Since the family is the basic unit of society, only if there is justice and democracy within the family can you possibly have justice and democracy in the wider society. In other words,

in mini skirts (this point has been exaggerated) but many of them unveiled. Far from being a black hole of gender apartheid, Afghanistan, although impoverished and backward, was still more progressive than many of its Muslim neighbors."[16] The fiction that cultural practices concerning women are immutable and untouchable is simply farce. The dynamic nature of gender practices must be monitored and archived, so that those who seek power by subjugating women cannot claim the legitimacy they crave.

THE STATE AS A DOUBLE-EDGED SWORD FOR WOMEN

In addition to the potential of CEDAW accession to make an important contribution to improving the status of women worldwide, the arena of state law is perhaps even more critical. While we have seen that laws on the books for women do not always translate into action on the ground, without the laws grassroots activities (detailed in chapter 6) will never ultimately succeed. As one Nepalese activist put it, "If we wash with a bucket of water and start from our feet, the water is wasted washing only our feet. But if we pour the water over our heads, we can wash our whole body."[17]

For women, the state is a double-edged sword: it can hurt them or it can defend them. Often, it does both; in fact, the record of the state concerning women is quite mixed. As we have seen, regimes struggling to gain legitimacy in traditional societies based on male dominance hierarchies will betray women, no matter how instrumental those women were in helping the new regime gain power. Other regimes are guilty of a studied neglect concerning women, even if fairly decent laws are on the books. The choice—for it is a choice—to not enforce equitable laws concerning women is also a betrayal of women by the state.

However, the crowning betrayals of women by the state must be identified as those that make women's bodies a tool of the state, overruling their inalienable human right to control their own bodies. The most salient examples of this are extreme pro-natalist and anti-natalist policies. Now, all regimes have some pro-natalist or anti-natalist policies; for example, the U.S. child tax credit can be seen as a pro-natalist policy. These mild policies are not what we have in mind; here we speak of forced childbearing and forced abortion/sterilization policies implemented by the state. To hijack women's bodies for the ends of the state is probably the most egregious harm a state can inflict. Some states, such as Japan during World War II and Romania during the Cold War, set a quota of

and into the full-term fetus to terminate it. The dead baby was extracted on September 9, 2000. When her husband, Yang, returned from his business trip, he rushed to the hospital to find Jin Yani purple and near death from blood loss. She spent 44 days in the hospital because of severe hemorrhaging. Now, she is infertile. . . . This incident is exceptional because Jin Yani and her husband, Yang, sued the Chinese government for the loss of their child and fertility. For the first time, a Beijing court agreed to hear the case. Later, a court in Qinhuangdao, Hebei province, ruled that certain officials should be replaced. This has not happened. Nor did the court offer any monetary compensation to Jin Yani or her husband. As of October of 2008, Jin Yani and Yang were living in hiding—not even their mothers know where they are. They cannot return to their village for fear that the cadres there will retaliate for the lawsuit.[23]

When we say that the state is a double-edged sword for women, this statement must be taken seriously. Unleashing the power of the state in the lives of women can have devastating consequences.

However, it can also not be denied that the state can be a powerful force for good for women. In the often very unequal balance of power within a household, the state, in some cases, can protect and nurture women in a manner that would otherwise never occur. In the language of the male dominance hierarchy, the state can become like a father or older brother to a woman—an extremely powerful father or older brother who is willing to hold her family, the woman's husband, and the men in the society accountable for what happens to her. The state can serve as a counterweight to the wishes and desires of her family, the husband and his family or, more generally, to the men of the society—and in some unmitigated male dominance societies, that counterweight can make an enormous and positive difference in the lives of women. The state has an important role in banking the incontinence of men, whether that incontinence manifests itself in household tyranny, financial sector recklessness, violent crime, unsustainably high fertility rates, or even imperial overreach. As we shall see, parity for women's voices in government is an important element in the state's ability to perform that role well.

STATE STRATEGIES

The diversity of strategies used by states to improve the status of women is impressive (table 5.2). The means by which state actors can create meaningful

TABLE 5.2 (*continued*)

STATE STRATEGY	VARIANTS
Make National Family Law Equitable	■ Establish a minimum age for marriage, preferably 18 ■ Grant equal right to divorce and access to custody for men and women ■ Prohibit polygyny ■ Equalize inheritance laws and property rights within marriage
Enact Pro-Women Legislation	■ Femicide laws ■ Asylum laws ■ Media image laws ■ Laws focusing on concrete enforcement measures
Change the Incentive Structures	■ Offer scholarships for girls ■ Pay for vaccinations for girls ■ Target development assistance to girls ■ Enforce pro-women laws, thus significantly increasing costs for those who would harm women
Include Women in Decision Making	■ Establish quotas for political representation ■ Facilitate greater access for female judges and attorneys ■ Create standards for gender composition of executive boards in private industry ■ Involve women in peace negotiations, *jirgas*, etc. ■ Promote greater presence of women on domestic police forces
Keep Caregiving Economically Rational	■ Equalize standards of living after divorce ■ Set standards of joint ownership of property in marriage ■ Address hiring and pay discrimination ■ Work toward proportional benefits for part-time workers ■ Provide pension benefits for unpaid caregiving ■ Provide paid maternity leave
R2PW	■ Fully implement UNSC and General Assembly resolutions that seek to improve the situation of women ■ Encourage regional IGO commitment to gender equity among member states ■ Monitor and track the situation of women within nations; this may involve gathering new statistics, conducting new research, etc. ■ Rank nations and sanction those with abominable records ■ Inventory best state practices to improve the situation of women ■ Redefine democracy to include whether a nation's women are valued, are secure, and have a voice

lives of women. Part of the problem is that women themselves do not know they are granted these rights; in some countries, high rates of illiteracy among women are part of the problem. But with a modest financial investment, states can rectify the situation. For example, Jordan has recently conducted a campaign to increase basic awareness of legal rights:

The campaign [in 2006] was launched by the Ministry of Political Development and Parliamentarian Affairs in cooperation with Mizan [an NGO]. "Our goal was to raise awareness about each person's legal rights and obligations," said Rula Haddadin, campaign manager at Mizan, also known as the Law Group for Human Rights. "Since the first days of the campaign, the number of phone calls we've received has increased considerably." In addition to a telephone hotline offering free legal advice, hundreds of billboards, CDs and pocket calendars were distributed in the capital, Amman, and at universities throughout the country aimed at informing citizens of their legal rights as enshrined in the constitution. Newspapers, television and radio spots were also used to spread the message.[26]

States could be even more creative in this endeavor; for example, they could emulate the work of Kristine Pearson and Lifeline Energy, which provides low-cost solar-powered and virtually indestructible radio/MP3 players to women in rural Africa. Radios and boom boxes are usually, in these cultures, the purview of men, as only men typically have the cash to spend on batteries. The provision of these "women's radios" allows women to tap into the larger world around them. One of the most important results, according to Pearson, is that women become cognizant of their legal rights for the first time, by listening in to women's radio programs. Furthermore, Pearson's organization can pre-load the MP3 player with files that not only promote literacy for women but also explain and summarize women's rights, so that every woman who has access to a radio will also have access to the information she needs to understand her legal rights.[27]

But there are further steps to be taken. Marilyn Waring has noted that the economic statistics that drive state policymaking completely omit any accounting of the unpaid labor contributions of women to the economy.[28] It is time for states to develop new measures of gross domestic product or gross domestic well-being that fully take into account the caretaking labor performed by women. When women are invisible in societal accounting, also rendered invisible to policymakers is an understanding of how policies may help or

still be crimes against humanity in times of peace? The court's ruling makes it possible to now raise this question in Sierra Leone society.

Discursive efforts could include state collaboration with media. For example, in Costa Rica, the Ministry of Women, in collaboration with women's NGOs, launched a series of "radio novellas" called *Love's Other Face*. Scriptwriters were hired to write entertaining half-hour chapters that would address issues of domestic violence and refute its normality and its legality.[36] In a sense, satellite television and the Internet have provided a "Radio Free Women" station, where women in nearly every land can see that it is possible for women to be treated as the equals of men. The discursive move is a powerful one that states can use to profound effect. For example, in an experiment run by Rob Jensen and Emily Oster, the provision to rural Indian communities of cable TV shows depicting educated, powerful women characters resulted in a significant decrease in the "aspiration gap" between male and female teenagers, as well as their parents. Just seeing a different and better life for women was sufficient to create new horizons for young women in these communities.[37]

HARVEST LOW-HANGING FRUIT

The government can also send messages to its citizenry through dealing with what we call here "low-hanging policy fruit." By banning a cultural practice that was formerly prevalent but is now comparatively rare, or banning a practice that is in its infancy but does not yet have broad-based societal support, the government can attempt to draw some brighter lines around the security of women.

An example of the former is premarital virginity testing. As this practice has fallen by the wayside in certain countries, some governments, including those of Jordan and Turkey, have taken the initiative to ban the practice outright, knowing there would be minimal backlash. An example of the latter is movement within several Western societies to ban the *niqab* and the burqa in public as inherently invisibilizing of women in the public space of society in a way that distinguishes this dress from the *chador* and *abaya*, as well as to ban sex-selective abortion. Obviously these practices are marginal in Western countries, but to ban something while the practices are still marginal also safeguards against future encroachment on the rights of women in these areas.[38]

Another variant of this strategy is to gradually increase the punishment for crimes against women, making a "lesser" crime into a "greater" crime. So, for

Physical Security of Women

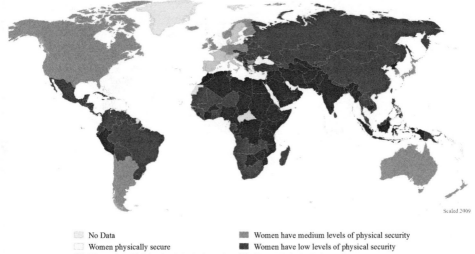

Scaled 2009

- No Data
- Women physically secure
- Women have high levels of physical security
- Women have medium levels of physical security
- Women have low levels of physical security
- Women lack physical security

MAP 1

Trafficking in Females

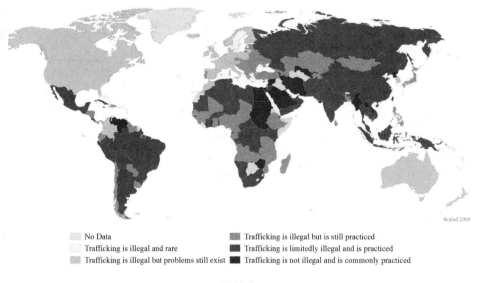

Scaled 2009

No Data

Trafficking is illegal and rare

Trafficking is illegal but problems still exist

Trafficking is illegal but is still practiced

Trafficking is limitedly illegal and is practiced

Trafficking is not illegal and is commonly practiced

MAP 3

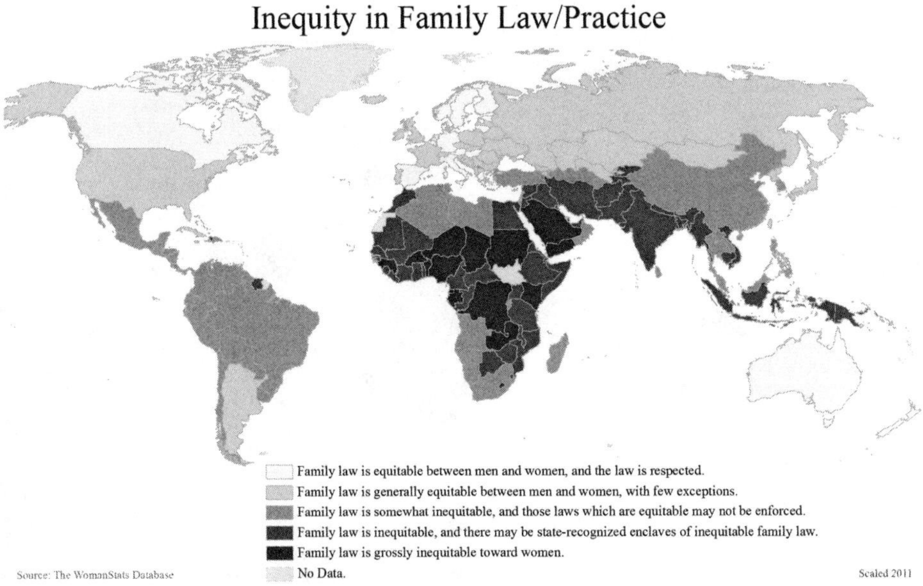

Inequity in Family Law/Practice

Family law is equitable between men and women, and the law is respected.
Family law is generally equitable between men and women, with few exceptions.
Family law is somewhat inequitable, and those laws which are equitable may not be enforced.
Family law is inequitable, and there may be state-recognized enclaves of inequitable family law.
Family law is grossly inequitable toward women.
No Data.

Source: The WomanStats Database

Scaled 2011

MAP 5

Discrepancy In Education

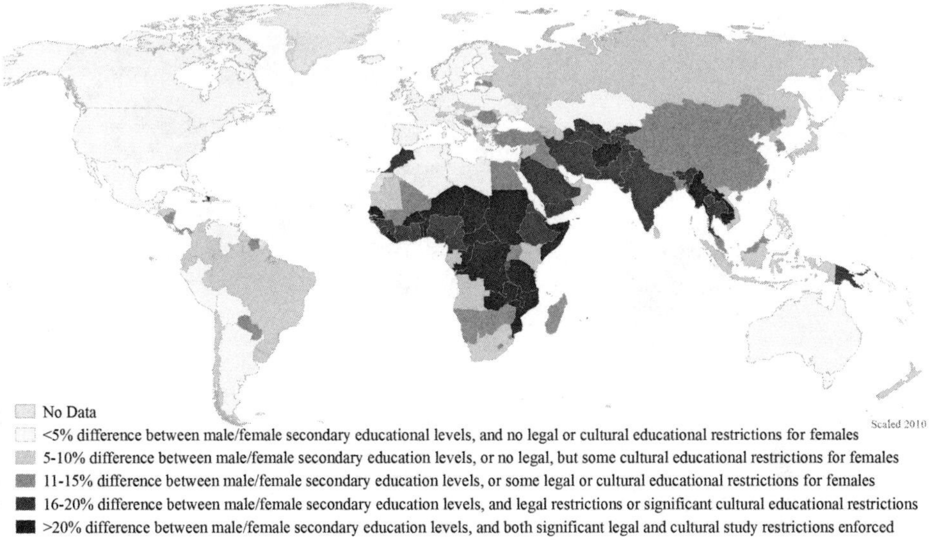

Scaled 2010

No Data

<5% difference between male/female secondary educational levels, and no legal or cultural educational restrictions for females

5-10% difference between male/female secondary education levels, or no legal, but some cultural educational restrictions for females

11-15% difference between male/female secondary education levels, or some legal or cultural educational restrictions for females

16-20% difference between male/female secondary education levels, and legal restrictions or significant cultural educational restrictions

>20% difference between male/female secondary education levels, and both significant legal and cultural study restrictions enforced

MAP 7

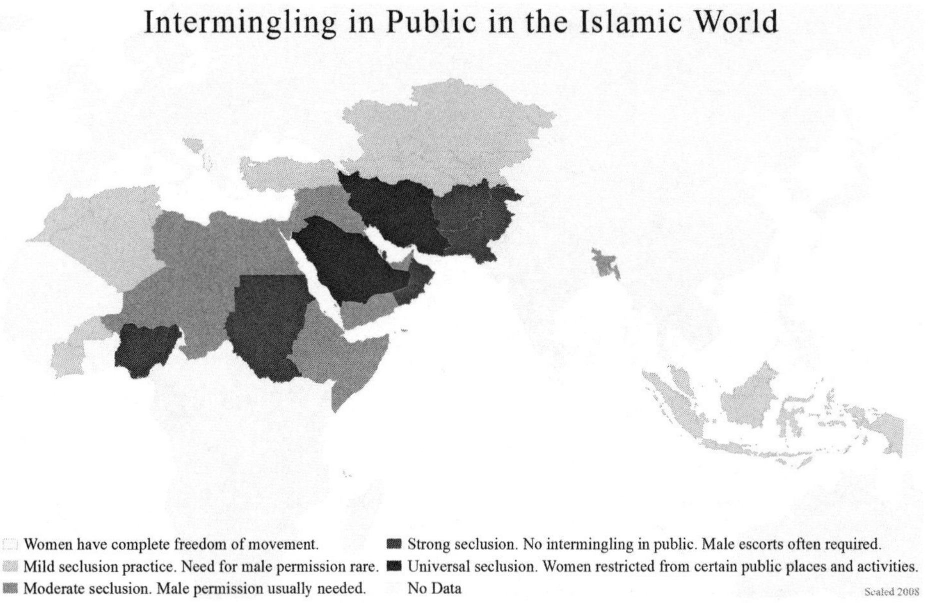

Intermingling in Public in the Islamic World

Women have complete freedom of movement.
Mild seclusion practice. Need for male permission rare.
Moderate seclusion. Male permission usually needed.

Strong seclusion. No intermingling in public. Male escorts often required.
Universal seclusion. Women restricted from certain public places and activities.
No Data

Scaled 2008

MAP 9

Discrepant Government Behavior Concerning Women

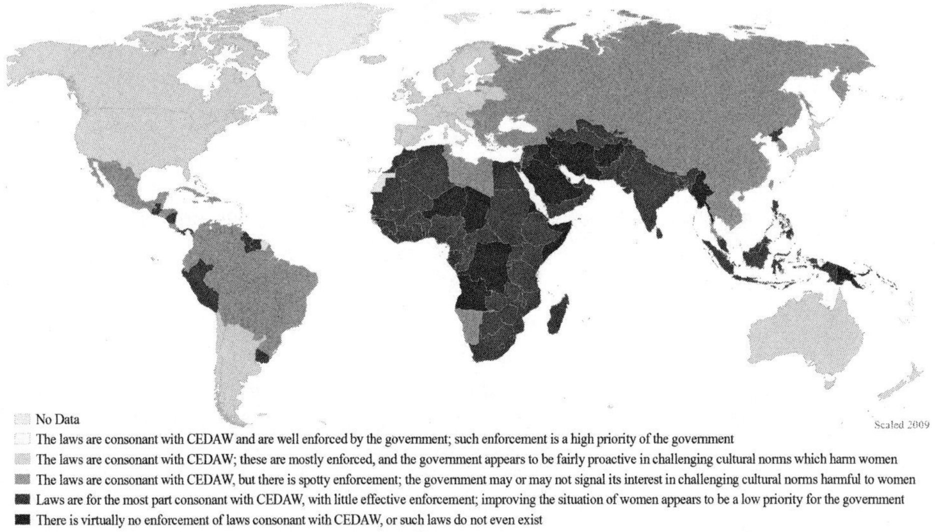

Scaled 2009

No Data
The laws are consonant with CEDAW and are well enforced by the government; such enforcement is a high priority of the government
The laws are consonant with CEDAW; these are mostly enforced, and the government appears to be fairly proactive in challenging cultural norms which harm women
The laws are consonant with CEDAW, but there is spotty enforcement; the government may or may not signal its interest in challenging cultural norms harmful to women
Laws are for the most part consonant with CEDAW, with little effective enforcement; improving the situation of women appears to be a low priority for the government
There is virtually no enforcement of laws consonant with CEDAW, or such laws do not even exist

MAP 11

enforced the ban.[41] The power of the powerful to steer public opinion can be effectively harnessed to improve the situation of women. We hope this situation is not reversed by the regime change in that nation.

It is also hard to overstate the crucial role played by King Mohammed VI of Morocco in protecting women of his country. A proclaimed descendant of the Prophet Mohammed, the king gave a historic speech on August 20, 1999, in which he stated, "How can society achieve progress, while women, who represent half the nation, see their rights violated and suffer as a result of injustice, violence, and marginalization, notwithstanding the dignity and justice granted them by our glorious religion?"[42] In 2004, the king shepherded an overhaul of family law in Morocco, giving women extraordinary rights compared with their sisters in other Islamic societies. (We detail those changes below.)

The emir of Kuwait, Shaikh Jabir al Ahmad, must also be singled out for special mention. Given the bravery of Kuwaiti women during Iraq's invasion of that country in 1990–1991 (when by and large the women stayed and fought, even in an armed resistance movement, while the men had to flee for their lives), after Kuwait's liberation, the emir began to argue that women could no longer be denied the full rights belonging to Kuwaiti citizens, including suffrage and the right to stand for office. Indeed, as early as 1999, the emir attempted to enact such legislation by decree, only to see his efforts nullified by the Kuwaiti parliament, manned by some of the most conservative (male) politicians in the country. He tried several times and failed each time. Finally in 2003, the emir went so far as to formally request that the Kuwaiti parliament honor him by acceding to his plea on this issue, which plea they rebuffed. The emir appointed two women to the Kuwaiti cabinet in early 2005, even though women still did not have the right to vote.

Finally in May 2005, through an intensive organized bottom-up effort featuring the largest and most inclusive public demonstration in Kuwaiti history, plus the added pressure from the emir, the Kuwaiti parliament granted women their suffrage. Shultziner and Tetreault argue that an important element in the passage of this act—which passage surprised both supporters and opponents—was the material inducements offered to members of parliament for their last-minute support, including increased salaries for government employees and increased pension payments, a price that may have totaled fifty million dollars.[43] When we speak, then, of the importance of state personalities in creating progress for women, we must acknowledge that rhetoric may have to be complemented by material pressure of both the carrot and the stick variety.

community of nations, bringing with it a full repertoire of both incentives and punishments at the bilateral and multilateral levels. State action to reduce maternal mortality need not try to uproot maternal health care systems already in place. For example, providing training for traditional birth attendants (TBAs), and providing them with LED lights powered by solar cells as well as inexpensive cell phones, can reduce maternal mortality even where hospitals are not nearby.[46]

Access to contraception is also part of nullifying the equation between sex and death for women, and the world community has enjoyed relative success in helping women obtain the means to control the reproduction of their own bodies. States must continue to subsidize the manufacture or import of contraception, as well as efforts to make it widely available and to provide training in how to use contraception, even to women in remote areas of the country.

Education of girls, as has been noted by many organizations and scholars, is one of the great keys to improving the situation of women. Educated women are better able to control what happens to their bodies, better able to avoid oppression in marriage, better able to safeguard their own health and the health of their children, better able to participate in the deliberations of human society. Many states have introduced innovative incentive systems to prod families to send girls to school. Successful initiatives include scholarships to waive school fees for girls, payments to families who send their girls to school and allow them time to complete their homework, the building of toilet facilities for girls at their schools, provision of sanitary supplies so that girls will not feel they have to miss school during menstruation, construction of schools closer to villages or provision of bicycles to girls so that they are not as vulnerable to attack while traveling to school, the training of female teachers, who are less likely to demand sex from girl students, and so forth. Again, the international community must be prepared to hold nations accountable where the literacy rate of girls is low, and to view such a statistic as tangible harm done to the peacefulness of the interstate system by the nation in question.

ENGAGE FORMAL AND INFORMAL JUDICIAL BODIES AT ALL LEVELS

One of the most effective steps to changing the law of the land is to open the way through judicial rulings. Appeal by judicial bodies to international treaties and covenants to which the nation-state is a party is an important element of such movement. As noted above, the Special Court in Sierra Leone has

of our discussion, to go back and confront this on religious grounds." . . . He did, explaining to the elders that nothing in the Quran prohibits a woman from talking with a man. In the end, no one was harmed.[51]

In another case in the Ivory Coast, women presented photographs of their lives, including depictions of domestic violence, to the village chief. The chief raised his arm. "I have heard your message," he said. "I do not want violence of any kind. If such violence goes on in this village, it must stop now." After the show he invited the photographers—who had formed an organization called Anouanze ("Unity")—to join his council of advisors. He invited all village women to attend village meetings. Overnight, cameras in hand, the women of Zatta village, who had never had a voice in public affairs, moved to the center of governance.[52]

Even "judicial systems" within the household itself must be considered a site of persuasion. When China got serious about its abnormal birth sex ratio, the government engaged in many educational outreach efforts. According to several observers, the most effective outreach was to the grandmothers—the mothers of the husbands of the pregnant women. These grandmothers have enormous power within the patrilocal household to force an abortion of a female fetus, and until the government makes them a special focus of education regarding the value of girl children, other educational efforts will have only suboptimal results.

PROHIBIT DEVELOPMENT OF INEQUITABLE FAMILY LAW ENCLAVES

As we noted in chapter 4, our research shows that inequitable family law is tightly correlated with high levels of violence against women. Nations that countenance enclaves of inequitable family law can expect higher rates of violence against women and lower levels of state peacefulness than states that refuse to allow such enclaves. The pressure on Western nations such as Canada, Australia, the UK, and others to permit such enclaves is rising. On the basis of our research findings, we strongly advocate for a complete prohibition of such enclaves, subordinating all households to equitable national family law standards.

Such prohibition demands that practices legal in other countries not be "imported" into a destination country where the practices are illegal. For example, nations such as the Netherlands recognize polygamous marriages if they were entered into within a country where polygamy is legal. This is

security. As political scientist Harry Eckstein has put it, "If any aspect of social life can directly affect government, it is the experience with authority that men have in other aspects of life."[55] We believe this applies first and foremost to family law.

As noted above, the nation of Morocco stands as an exemplar in this regard. While Westerners erroneously believe that women's legal rights are incompatible with Islamic law, King Mohammed VI has proven otherwise. The Moudawana, or Family Law, passed in 2004 provides many outstanding examples of how a state can "get" the linkage between the security of women and the security of states. Examples include:

- Legal age of marriage is eighteen for both sexes
- Polygamy is severely constrained, to the point of practical impossibility
- A judge must handle all divorces, even *talaq* divorces in which all that is required is for the husband to say, "I divorce you" three times.
- Children can choose with which parent they wish to live at age fifteen
- Grandchildren from daughters inherit in the same way as grandchildren from sons
- Property is divided equitably after divorce; standard of living for both parties should be similar after divorce
- The duty of a wife to obey her husband is abolished in return for the wife's equal responsibility to support the household
- A divorced wife may retain custody of children even if she remarries

From the point of view of anthropological research, it is the first two items that are the most significant. As we have seen, ensuring that girls are not married at puberty, but several years afterward, and ensuring that polygamy is virtually abolished are two vitally important elements of family law that increase national security. Egypt adds another stipulation, which is also commendable: it forbids marriages between men and women where the age difference is greater than twenty-five years.[56] Also important would be state initiatives to equalize inheritance, especially of land, between male and female heirs, as well as measures to discourage patrilocality, which make brides exceedingly vulnerable to abuse and violence.

We encourage the international community to develop a set of benchmarks in family law, educating and encouraging nations to see equitable family law, and its enforcement in practice, as part of the bedrock of national and international security.

are not stopped then I fear a movement for enforcement of true Islamic sharia would be launched throughout the country."[61]

Interestingly, while Saudi Arabia inches toward sixteen as the legal age of marriage, Yemen, to the south, is facing stiff opposition in a similar quest, despite horrific cases of young girls dying from intercourse and childbirth after being married as young as age eight to fully adult men. One influential cleric insisted he would gather a million signatures against any legislation that would forbid child marriage. He deemed those supporting a rise in the marriage age as apostates.[62] The weak Yemeni government would rather not upset the micro-level patriarchs whose acquiescence it needs to govern, and it seems likely that the little girls of Yemen will be left with no protection.

CHANGE THE INCENTIVE STRUCTURES

The state has the power to alter the web of incentives and disincentives in which households must operate—and it can do this to the benefit of women. As we have noted previously, some states pay families to send their daughters to school.

Other examples abound. For example, the problem of abnormal birth sex ratios has plagued both China and India. Each state has sought to alter incentive structures for families. In China, a new "Care for Girls" program was launched, which waives school fees for rural girls and guarantees a (small) pension for families that have only daughters. China has also promoted uxorilocal marriages, where a groom marries into his bride's family, supports his in-laws in their old age (something not normally done when an only child, a daughter, goes to live with her husband's parents), and does not pass his surname on to his children. Such families may receive land grants, and the government will build them a house as well.

India has a new pilot program operative in states with the worst sex ratios. If a family has a daughter, they will be paid to keep her with an initial grant of money, and then be paid for various important events, such as vaccinations and school attendance. Then, if the girl reaches the age of eighteen, has graduated from school, and is not yet married, the government will pay several thousand dollars toward her wedding expenses (dowries are technically illegal in India).

Making investment in girls' health and well-being profitable for families is one way in which the state can alter circumstances for the better for women. Furthermore, as we have seen, through proactive enforcement of

ing the quota system to the state and national governments: the upper house of the national legislature has already approved such legislation.

Ironies abound. While the United States has one of the lowest levels of female representation in the national legislature, the Americans ensured that both of the countries they recently invaded—Afghanistan and Iraq—enshrined quotas for women. Bulgaria now has one of the highest representations in Europe in its executive branch, but the reason for it is that the charismatic male prime minister finds women more pliable to work with than men.[64]

Each society seems to walk the path toward greater female representation in its own idiosyncratic way. So, for example, Saudi Arabia has announced that female lawyers may now appear in court—but only in family court, and only to represent female clients. Egypt, on the other hand, refuses to allow women to serve the Supreme Judicial Council, though they may otherwise be judges. Norway not only has quotas for women in government but also has quotas for women on the boards of publicly traded corporations. Thirty-six percent of the personnel on such boards are women; the highest percentage in the world, and the legislated minimum is 40 percent.[65] Fiji has recently legislated that the minister with the gender portfolio be included as a member of the National Security Council. By government mandate, more than two million women are now involved in the local panchayats of India, bringing water, electricity, and girls' schools to some of the most remote areas of that country.[66]

It is not only at the highest levels that women must be included and visible. When women are visibly making a contribution in public and on the ground, the culture begins to change. One example of this is the Daughters of Iraq unit formed to help combat suicide terrorism in that country. These women—a total of 130 have graduated thus far—are part of the Iraqi security forces, and they are responsible for searching women for explosives. "The women's proudest moment came in March, when thousands of people from across Baghdad, including the country's Shiite prime minister, converged in Adhamiya to celebrate the prophet Muhammad's birthday. The Daughters of Iraq were out in force, patting down women as they approached Abu Hanifa, the city's most revered Sunni mosque. 'A lot of women were happy to see the local women there to protect them,' Dulaimi said. 'They were hugging and kissing us and giving us Pepsis.'"[67] Lamentably, the Daughters of Iraq are an invention of the Americans, and the Iraqi government has no intention of retaining them once the Americans leave. Indeed, when the Iraqi government took control, it stopped paying the women, and many quit to seek paid employment.[68]

Power, tempered by the wisdom and restraint of responsibility, is the foundation of a just society. But with too little responsibility, power turns to tyranny. And with too little power, responsibility becomes exploitation. Yet in every country in the world, power and responsibility have become unbalanced and unhitched, distributed unequally between men and women. . . . The penalties of women's too-great burden of responsibility and their too-small slice of power . . . are hardship, sickness, hunger, even famine. But the penalties of man's disproportionate share of the world's power (without the intimate day-to-day knowledge of the effects of that power, or the responsibility for ensuring that the basic needs of the household are met) are just as great.

Of course, not all men are tyrants or despots and not all women are martyrs to duty and hard work. But masculine and feminine social roles have tilted the majority of men and women in those directions.[69]

It is time, then, for power and responsibility to be married by states. Caregiving must count—really count—in the perspective of national governments.

IMPLEMENT A STATE RESPONSIBILITY TO PROTECT WOMEN (R2PW)

As of 2001, the world began to recognize that states have a Responsibility to Protect (R2P) their citizens, an idea that the UN General Assembly endorsed in 2005. The international community identifies three pillars of R2P:

- States have primary responsibility to protect their populations from genocide, war crimes, ethnic cleansing, and crimes against humanity.
- The international community must commit to provide assistance to States in building capacity to protect their populations from these and assist them both before crises and after crises have broken out.
- It is the responsibility of the international community to take timely and decisive action to prevent and halt atrocities when a State is manifestly failing to protect its populations. The international community has the obligation to intervene at first diplomatically, and as a last result, with force.

It is time to recognize that R2P includes R2PW—a Responsibility to Protect Women. It is time to put the situation of women in the nations of the world as one of the foremost issues facing the international community today. It is time for the UN Security Council and General Assembly to hold nations

according to their level of R2PW. There is simply too much that we haven't bothered to try to know. For example, according to Donald Steinberg, deputy president of the International Crisis Group,

[I]n pressing for UN action to halt the latest round of violence in eastern DRC in November, a Congolese women's declaration at the Association for Women's Rights in Development could refer only to "thousands of raped women and girls," with no greater specificity. Similarly, an otherwise powerful letter to Secretary-General Ban Ki-moon from the NGO Working Group on Women, Peace and Security could say only that the 66 women treated for rape in Kanyabayonga in North Kivu "represent only a fraction of the crimes of sexual violence being committed throughout the region." [A]dditional authoritative data from the ground are essential in to meeting [*sic*] the "threshold of credibility" needed to build political will, providing measurement tools to assess new and on-going efforts at prevention, developing specific provisions and programs to maximize our efforts, and ensuring that the critical mass of officials from international organizations, governments and civil society that came together to adopt Resolution 1820 will remain together in the face of shrinking resources that will require tough trade-offs.[74]

We have already noted the need for gender-disaggregated statistics to be produced by national governments; we also need the infrastructure to mandate the phenomena studied by national statistical bureaus. In particular, we need more and better statistics on violence against women, especially violence within the home. Excellent frameworks for the monitoring and collection of such data do exist,[75] but what is missing is the political and international will to implement them. Such frameworks must be multivariate — after all, if you knew only that the representation of women in South Africa's national legislature was one of the highest in the world, would that compensate for not knowing that South Africa has by far the highest rape rate in the world?

Such a multivariate ranking of R2PW not only would serve as a mechanism for action against states that are egregious in their negligence concerning their obligations, but also could help to focus state efforts in areas of particular concern. For example, while most view Sweden as a haven for women, reports indicate that levels of domestic violence in Sweden have spiraled upward in recent years.[76] A detailed and comprehensive analysis of R2PW-relevant measures could be useful in spotting such problems early.

would be in a position to apply sanctions—yes, sanctions—to those states that failed in their R2PW.[77]

A FARTHER SHORE

Should the world ever take seriously the concept that the two halves of humanity must be true and equal partners for humankind to flourish, we see a farther shore to which we might aspire to travel. Glimpses of that shore are visible even now.

For example, the 2009 Nobel Women's Initiative Conference issued an extraordinary statement:

We call upon all states and multilateral institutions to recognize that the democratization process is incomplete, and does not end with elections. No country or society can claim to be democratic when the women who form half its citizens are denied their right to life, to their human rights and entitlements, and to safety and security. Despite this, we women have made extraordinary efforts to democratize the institutions of society that frame our lives and the well-being of all humanity—the family, the community, clan, tribe, ethnic or religious group, political, legal, economic, social and cultural structures, and the media and communications systems. But our search for justice is continually overwhelmed by the violence perpetrated upon us, by the exploitation and colonization of our bodies, our labor, and our lands; by militarization, war and civil conflict; by persistent and increasing poverty; and by environmental degradation. All of these forces affect us, and our children, far more severely and in unique ways. We know that democracy that comes from the heart is not the rule of the majority, but safeguards dissent and difference with equal rights, and fosters a culture of peace. We are in search of democracy that transforms not just our lives, but all society—and we will not be silenced until it is achieved in every part of the world.[78]

Perhaps it is time to redefine the very term "democracy," to insist that its definition include only those states that have made the greatest strides toward gender equality. Perhaps, then, we should make the world safe for this understanding of democracy, reorganizing IGO and alliance commitments according to one's position in the global clash of gender civilizations. Maybe

6

WINGS OF NATIONAL AND INTERNATIONAL RELATIONS, PART TWO

Effecting Positive Change Through Bottom-Up Approaches

THE WOUNDING OF OUR world's women can seem overwhelming. Even well-intended top-down efforts to provide women with physical security, equity in family law, and opportunities to participate in social and political decision making face many obstacles and may take time to make a difference on the ground. While every top-down approach must be pursued, we cannot simply wait for large organizations and governments to act. Furthermore, top-down efforts will almost certainly be more effective if there is a mirroring effort at the social level. We must further the cause at every level of society, including at the grassroots level, where we can work to protect one woman, and then another, and then another, until more and more women benefit from our efforts. It is reported that Mother Teresa once said, "If I look at the mass, I will never act. If I look at the one, I will."[1]

Bottom-up efforts to improve the status of women are perhaps most needed in countries of the world where government leadership is openly patriarchal and resistant to change. But even governments that proclaim their commitment to improving conditions for women often do not give that commitment the priority it deserves, as they are slow to enact policies and laws that would really make a difference for women. In recent years, some individuals have taken the matter into their own hands and joined their efforts with those of others, creating a groundswell of successful bottom-up work to bring about small changes wherever they can.[2] Women, frequently in concert with men, are starting to make a difference, and their voices are beginning to be heard. While gendered microaggression and structural inequities, as outlined in chapters 1 and 2, appear daunting, the agency of women can never be fully repressed; as we shall see, it finds ever new and creative means of expression.

On the day of the lavish wedding with live music, two thousand guests, food, and a dowry of two televisions, two home theater sets, two refrigerators, two air conditioners, and one car, the groom's family demanded an illegal cash payment of $25,000. When Nisha's father said he couldn't pay, the Dalals erupted in anger, and an outbreak ensued between the two families. In the midst of the chaos, Nisha reached for her cell phone and called the police. When the police arrived, they encouraged the families to proceed with the ceremony, but Nisha refused, saying, "If they treated [my father] so badly, they probably would have done the same to me, or worse." In fact, in India it is not uncommon for resentment over small dowries to be connected to suspicious "kitchen fires," which have been responsible for the deaths of several thousand newly married women each year.

Thus, the wedding was embarrassingly canceled, the groom and his mother were arrested, and Nisha became the face of the modern Indian woman. She was hailed for her courageous decision in a situation that often brings shame and mockery upon the bride's family. Shortly after this single decision, similar stories of brave brides and greedy grooms surfaced, with the women following Nisha's example. Six months later she married a computer hardware engineer—*without* a dowry.[4]

Pervinder Kaur arrived in New York as a bride from India to be married to a wealthy man. Instead, vulnerable and knowing very little about America, she was trapped as a prisoner by her new in-laws. They forbade her from making friends outside the family, and her husband beat her and tried to coerce her to turn over money. She had the presence of mind to take a single step and make two phone calls. The first call was to the police, who sent her to the hospital. And the second call was to a support group, Sakhi ("female friend"), that was run by volunteers who help women, one at a time. The women are usually from India, Bangladesh, Pakistan, Nepal, and the Caribbean. Sakhi is part of a growing movement across the country that confronts taboo social issues and hidden abuses in immigrant families. They teach the women about their rights and how to exercise them, help them find safe places to live, provide language assistance and legal advice, and even accompany them to court or interviews with the police. Pervinder recounts the comfort she found in discovering a familiar culture. "They spoke so nicely to me. They talked in my language. Until then, I could not talk about it, what had happened. I always started to cry."[5]

Gang rapes sanctioned by tribal councils as a form of honor revenge are not uncommon in Pakistan, and any self-respecting woman is expected to

cides to go out and work, it is often frowned upon, even if she is doing it to support her family."

One woman who has benefited from the center is Horeya Abo Gohar, whose husband died thirteen years ago, leaving her to raise five children. She explained, "I have learned so much from coming here. It has taken me a long time but I have finally realized that whatever a man does I can do too . . . [T]his center gave me the strength to understand that. In the beginning I thought I would not be able to do anything with my life . . . but last year I found the strength to open my own business as a child minder, and now I take care of other women's children so that they can go out to work."[9]

One of the most stirring cases in recent years illustrating the power of one step is that of Nujood Ali, a ten-year-old Yemeni girl who was married in 2007 at age nine without her consent to a man in his thirties. After her husband forced himself upon her, beat her, and took her out of school, she took the amazing step of hailing a taxi for the first time in her young life. She had heard that judges in courts granted divorces, and she was determined to see a judge. After arriving at the court building, she waited in the hallway, asking to see a judge. The judge was shocked by her story, and he made a momentous decision both for himself and for the country: "I am going to help you."[10] Still another judge took her into his home to protect her, and a female lawyer, Shada Nasser, agreed to represent her; her divorce was granted. Nujood recently won *Glamour* magazine's award for Woman of the Year. She wants to become a lawyer and is helping to raise funds to fight child marriage in Yemen. All of this came from one little girl having the courage to raise her hand to hail a taxi.[11]

In each of these instances, a single individual made one decision—to ask a question, to refuse to give in to social pressure, to reach out for help, or to help others. Such small acts of prosocial behavior significantly affected other women around that individual, and the circumstances in which those women lived started to improve. No act to redress the suffering of women is too small; take one small step wherever you can.

WHEREVER POSSIBLE, ENGAGE OTHERS IN YOUR CAUSE, SPREAD THE WORD, AND ORGANIZE

Having been raped when she was six years old, Betty Makoni understands the devastation that comes from such a traumatizing experience, and she works unceasingly to campaign for protection for young girls in Zimbabwe. The

is asked to influence ten others, in this way symbolically linking up with the 50 million "missing women" in the region.[15]

"The two messages that are repeatedly communicated are that women are no less valuable than men and that violence against them is unacceptable." It is the position of this movement that deeply entrenched attitudes can be changed only by many people working together. Eighteen-year-old Kavitha of Chowdaripatti village, Nalagonda district, Andhra Pradesh, India, says, "Before becoming part of the campaign, I was accustomed to remaining silent at home and accepting everything I was told. But now I request my father to accommodate my mother's needs and hear her out so that her opinions can also be taken into account. I have been explaining the contents of the campaign communication material to people in the village in the hope that men in other families will do the same as my father. I do not know whether I will succeed but I am trying."

Many other examples of changes in attitudes suggesting that violence is less tolerated have been credited to the campaign. In Nepal, a group of boys who had been enlisted as Change Makers in the We Can campaign and were wearing their We Can T-shirts saw some girls being harassed. The boys rushed to intervene and persuaded the troublemakers not to continue in such behavior. Other boys who had not worn their T-shirts ran home to put them on and returned to the scene. In such small ways, change is beginning, and the organization of individual efforts to bring about change in the acceptability of violence against women increases the power to transform social attitudes.

USE TECHNOLOGY TO AMPLIFY YOUR MESSAGE

One of the more visible accounts of using technology to speak out to thousands and thousands is that of Rania al-Baz, a popular Saudi TV host. During her segments on a show called *The Kingdom This Morning*, she would wear colorful *hijabs* and never cover her face. Her life all changed on one evening in April 2004, when her violent husband pounded her face into a marble floor until he thought she was dead while their five-year-old son watched. As her husband drove to dispose of her body, she started to regain consciousness, so he dropped her off at an emergency room, saying she had been in an accident. She lay in a coma for four days. While she was recovering, her father took photos of her disfigured face, which had thirteen factures.

Knowing that in Saudi Arabia domestic violence was commonly carried out but seldom talked about, Rania decided to go public. Two weeks after

foreign broadcasting companies, including some Arab-based stations like al-Jazeera out of Qatar and Dubai TV. Two examples of such programs are a 2008 debate between a Saudi cleric and a Saudi women's rights activist on marriage, guardians, driving, and other women's issues,[20] and *The Oprah Winfrey Show*, which did not tackle Islamic-specific issues but certainly introduced new and interesting ideas to women. From its first broadcast in Saudi Arabia in 2004, *Oprah* was an instant hit and became the highest-rated English-language (with Arabic subtitles) program among women age twenty-five and under. According to Katherine Zoepf of the *New York Times*, "Ms. Winfrey provides many young Saudi women with new ways of thinking about the way local taboos affect their lives along with a variety of issues including childhood sexual abuse and coping with marital strife. Above all, Ms Winfrey assures her viewers that no matter how restricted or even abusive their circumstances may be, they can take control in small ways and create lives of value, and she helps them 'find meaning in their . . . existence.'"[21]

Film, too, is challenging ideas in closed societies and is being used as a way to bring about change. A few years ago Tunisian filmmaker Kalthoum Bornaz considered the issue of inheritance rights for women in her movie *Shtar Mahaba* (Half the Love). The story focuses on twins, Selim (male) and Selima (female). When Selima was still young, she learned about Islamic inheritance laws and asked her father if her getting only half of the amount her brother got meant that her father loved her only half as much. When opposition arose against the film, director Bornaz countered that she had made the movie not to challenge inheritance practices but as a way "to discuss the issue of inheritance from a humane and social perspective."[22] Filmmakers in Iran also are beginning to see film as way to bring about change. Female documentary filmmaker Mahnaz Mohammadi explained that "we make films to change the status quo."[23]

One such female filmmaker is Tahmineh Milani, who makes movies about the violation of women's rights and hopes thereby "to create positive changes" in society.[24] A partial list of some of the movies she has created shows her passion for portraying the injustices that women face in modern-day Iran.[25] *Two Women* (1999) focuses on the hurdles, including domestic violence, that two female architectural students encounter in trying to fulfill their dreams. *Vakonesh Panjom* (The Fifth Reaction, 2003) explores the issue of custodial rights through the story of a widow who struggles against her father-in-law to maintain custody of her children and ownership of her home. The more recent *Payback*, released in 2010 after a ban of three years by Iran's Ministry of

out! It's just not appropriate, especially here in our culture."[32] In an effort to have the law enforced and to get women working in lingerie shops, college lecturer Reem Assad turned to Facebook, where she created a site titled in Arabic "Women's Undergarments for Women Only." The site, with comments in both Arabic and English, has over 5,700 members, and the law is now being more consistently enforced.[33] Also in Saudi Arabia, MySpace was used by an all-girl rock band. Although they are forbidden from playing in public, they are able to post their music, which can then be downloaded by young Saudis.[34]

Web sites and blogs are other digital tools increasingly used in the Islamic world. In Iran, for example, women mobilized to change laws on marriage, divorce, adultery, and polygyny by organizing the Campaign for One Million Signatures. Because of governmental suppression, it is increasingly difficult to collect signatures through traditional methods of canvassing. This online effort centered on its Web site (www.we-change.org), but the movement has met with strong governmental opposition, including the jailing of several score of its members, prohibiting other members from leaving the country, and the blocking of its Web site more than eighteen times. Still, it has had an impact. One of its founders, Susan Tahmasebi, notes: "We feel we achieved a great deal even though we are faced with security charges. No one is accusing us of talking against Islam. No one is afraid to talk about more rights for women anymore. This is a big achievement."[35]

A mother of three and postgraduate student who is also the anonymous author of Saudiwoman's weblog uses the Web to disseminate her writings, many of which deal with women's issues.[36] In various posts she has condemned the arranged marriage of a sixty-five-year-old man to an eleven-year-old girl and attacked the Saudi gender apartheid that is found in all sectors of society, including women's sections in government ministries that are housed inside buildings and accessed through back doors. In several posts she calls for change in the driving laws. While this blog is perhaps limited in its influence, the number of positive comments on it shows that technology facilitates the discussion on women's issues and that they are of interest to many.

Silence Speaks is an international digital storytelling initiative offering a safe environment for telling stories that too often remain unspoken. Participants from all over the world share and bear witness to tales of struggle and courage, resulting in short digital videos. These first-person stories aim to challenge media legacies by ensuring that workshop participants, not producers, have primary control over what is shared and how events and people

sible for women to take up the sport of golf again, and they are doing so in increasing numbers.[38]

Sometimes the best way to pursue change might be to seriously and continuously prepare yourself for the day when opportunity will knock. Who would have thought that one day women would be designing mosques or that they would be able to worship in an inviting space? In Turkey, with its long tradition of magnificent mosque architecture, a woman interior designer has shaken things up with a new mosque, whose interior she designed with "women in mind." The *mihrab*, indicating the direction of prayer, is bright turquoise and in the shape of a seashell, and the *mimbar* (pulpit) is made of acrylic rather than of the traditional wood or stone. Perhaps most importantly, unlike most mosques where women are segregated into poorly lit, partitioned-off back sections and balconies, this mosque positions the women's section in a well-lit open balcony with a nice view of the beautiful central chandelier.[39] For many years to come, women will be psychologically uplifted and better able to worship in such an inspiring setting, never before available to them. Fortunately, one woman prepared herself well long before she was given an opportunity to use her training in such a beneficial way for women.

Several scholars have noted that the most impressive progress for women has occurred when women stood ready and organized to press for their demands during times of unforeseen upheaval. As noted in chapter 5, when the emir of Kuwait was able to bring pressure again on parliament in 2005 to extend suffrage to women, the parliament was considering a partial suffrage in municipal elections only. Sensing that the moment was now or never, women's groups reached out to other groups in society and organized the largest demonstration in Kuwaiti history, creating the momentum for the emir to push through full and complete suffrage for women in a whirlwind of events. If women had not been ready when the moment came, they might never have achieved their goal.[40]

Civil or interstate war, or irregular regime transitions, can also provide opportunities for women, if women are ready to seize them. At these times of upheaval, if women are organized and tenaciously push their cause, remarkable progress can be achieved. We can see this dynamic in Rwanda, where organized women's groups stood ready to press for gains in the wake of the genocide of 1994 and the subsequent reconstruction of the government. Rwanda now boasts the highest percentage of women legislators of any country in the world—more than half of the legislators in the country are women.

occur over time. In fact, a saying has emerged that captures a growing acceptance of change: "Even the Masai are wearing underwear now." The father
of one student, Christine Shuaka, suddenly announced after school one day
that she was to be married. He dropped talk of marriage, however, when he
was able to see that she was doing well in school and has said that it is very
important for her to be educated.[41]

When change for women does not come because it is impeded by culture
or religion, some women have chosen to protest, resist, or challenge the system. One of the more poignant accounts of standing up for what is in the best
interest of women and the future of their country comes from a girls' school
in Afghanistan. We mentioned the story of Shamsia Husseini and her sister in
chapter 2. As they were walking to school, some men who objected to education for girls sprayed them with acid. Scars, jagged and discolored, now spread
across Shamsia's eyelids and most of her left cheek. These days, her vision
goes blurry, making it hard for her to read. Although the attack was meant
to terrorize the girls into staying home, it appears to have completely failed.
Nearly all of the wounded girls returned to the Mirwais School, including
Shamsia, whose face was so badly burned that she had to be sent abroad for
treatment. Perhaps even more remarkable, nearly every other female student
in this deeply conservative community returned as well—about 1,300 in all.
Only a couple of dozen girls regularly miss school now; three of them are girls
who were injured in the attack.[42] Never give up.

THERE ARE ALWAYS CULTURALLY SENSITIVE WAYS TO IMPROVE CONDITIONS FOR WOMEN; REDEFINE HONOR AS PROMOTING PROGRESS FOR WOMEN

Some of the most effective efforts in facilitating women's progress and fur-
thering peace require that the agents of change build upon the cultural and
religious roots of those with whom they are working—even in cases where
one is working with one's own fellow citizens. Whether we speak of the West,
the East, or any other region of the world, culture is a powerful force and
must be respected. When this approach is used, improvements for women
are viewed as being compatible with local values, and when at least some
values are shared, some predictable conflicts can be avoided and progress thus
expedited. Consider the story of Isnino Shuriye, who was revered throughout
northeastern Kenya as an expert female genital cutter. She started out as a
young apprentice who held down the legs of girls while her mother performed

In Turkey, women have sought greater rights to participate within the organizational structure of Islam. Turkey's religious institutions, to their credit, have taken these requests seriously and have acted to effect progress. They have appointed hundreds of women as preachers (*vaizes*) and as deputies to muftis with the task of monitoring the work of imams in local mosques, particularly as it relates to women. Zuleyha Seker, one of eighteen *vaizes* in Istanbul, explained that she does not give sermons or lead prayers; her main duty is to teach religion classes for women. She said, "In the past, [women] believed anything told to them by their older brother, father, or teacher. But as they are becoming more educated, they are coming up with more questions. We need new answers for new questions." Seker holds a degree in theology and with these new opportunities to teach women, she and others are in unique positions to strengthen women from within the Islamic structure.[45]

Sometimes traditions can be reinterpreted in a way that allows progress for women. Rather than pitting culture in a zero sum game against the rights of women, activists look for a win-win reinterpretation of a cultural practice. For example, though dowry is illegal in India, it is still widely practiced. However, some elite families have asserted that the money they spend on a high-quality college education (and even postgraduate degrees) for their daughters is in fact the dowry they provide to the groom's family. In this case, rather than denying the practice of dowry, they are reinterpreting dowry itself to value educational investment in women.

Whenever better practices for women can be seen as compatible with already accepted theological and cultural foundations, people should not be asked to give up their roots but rather to build upon them. This approach validates core concepts of the self-image and at the same time helps individuals transcend misconceptions with newer, more equitable ways to view women. In a way, roots are necessary for wings.

The work of Kwame Anthony Appiah is noteworthy in this regard. Appiah suggests that invoking the deep honor/shame emotions and simultaneously redefining what honor means is what leads to the swiftest, surest change for the better. In his book *The Honor Code: How Moral Revolutions Happen*, Appiah recounts how Confucian scholar Kang Youwei, through interaction with foreigners, came to feel ashamed of the practice of foot-binding for women. Appiah writes, "In 1898, Kang sent a memorandum to the emperor. 'All countries have international relations, and they compare their political institutions with one another,' he began, 'so that if one commits the slightest error, the

In Amman, Jordan, the mobility of women has been given a boost by the installation of new flat sidewalks lined with park benches. According to the urban planners who designed them, the sidewalks were viewed as powerful tools of social planning, tearing down walls between rich and poor, helping a city bereft of an identity to develop a sense of place and ownership. While perhaps not initially intended as such, the new pedestrian pathways and benches have also provided an acceptable way for women to get out and about. Twenty-year-old Reem al-Hambali explained, "If you're a girl and you're just hanging out on a regular street or sitting on a sidewalk, it's considered inappropriate. Everyone will look at you and ask, 'Why is this girl sitting there?' But here it's okay. We can sit here and it's normal."[49]

Sheema Kerma of Pakistan has used theater as a creative way to teach people about women's rights. She resisted great pressure in order to revive theater and dance when everything was banned during General Zia ul-Haq's regime. She did so because she believes that art is one of the most powerful ways to communicate with others and present them with new ideas. Sheema founded Tehrik-e-Niswan (Women's Movement) and has staged plays that consider such forbidden topics as domestic violence, rape, child molestation, and education for girls. Her work is often met with opposition and threats. A few years ago, Sheema's troupe planned to perform a play about girls' education in a large slum in Karachi. The men of the community insisted that they screen the play before any women were allowed to see it. Given the message of the show, the men chose to not allow it. "The decision should have made me sad," Sheema says. "But it only reinforced that this medium is so powerful that people are scared of it. Those men thought the play would inspire or incite women to think for themselves—and that's what we want." In spite of all of her creative efforts, Sheema admits that there is growing resistance to the arts. She laments, "For years, I've been performing in all corners of Pakistan, and no one has shut us down. But the mullahs [clerics] in the crowd are growing in number. I don't know if theater can defeat the fashion of fundamentalism."[50]

While Ann Jones was a volunteer with the International Rescue Committee, she went from country to country on the committee's Gender-Based Violence Unit with a project titled "A Global Crescendo: Women's Voices from Conflict Zones." This project was designed to document all aspects of women's daily lives, including widespread sexual exploitation and wife beating, in order to help them talk together about their problems and create their own agenda for change. The women were given digital cameras and worked

logic. Moudhi is now reportedly pressing for "donkey parking" at office buildings and shops!

INVOLVE MEN IN YOUR INITIATIVES

Men still hold the lion's share of structural power and voice within human societies. Sometimes one's efforts can be much more successful if men are involved with the initiative. It may be that men in patriarchal societies listen only to other eminent men, and what they say will be men's primary source of encouragement to treat women more equitably and humanely.

In the fall of 2009 history was made when for the first time a Palestinian female soccer team competed on the international level by playing a team from Jordan. For team manager Rukayya Takrori, the game was more than just a game. She explained, "In our culture Palestinian women work side by side with the men in the fields and factories. They fight together, demonstrate together. Sometimes she takes the place of the man because he is in jail or is in the mountains, hiding." She then concluded: "Palestinian women can do everything—even football."

The women's team was the brainchild of a man—Jibril Rajoub, the president of the Palestinian Football Association and the former chief of a feared security organization in the West Bank. In that position of importance, he encouraged the hiring of women in all departments, something that he boasts "erased forever the idea of ladies being only secretaries." When he took over the command of the football association in 2008, he created a women's soccer league. In their first game, the women played before ten thousand cheering West Bank fans, one-quarter of them men. Most of the women played bareheaded, but one Palestinian team member and a few from the Jordanian team wore *hijabs* while playing. Without a man like Rajoub throwing his support and creativity behind the team, we cannot imagine how such an event would ever have happened.[53]

When men change, they can describe the process of change for other men in a way that women cannot. Women for Women International launched its Men's Leadership Program in one province of the Democratic Republic of Congo where there was pervasive gender-based violence and deeply entrenched barriers regarding gender roles and authority. Educating influential community members has been successful in creating more women's rights advocates among Congolese men. One man describes the program as opening his eyes and giving him a new life. He had previously considered his wife

When asked why a man would take on the cause of women's rights, Bassam explained, "Trying to stop violence and discrimination against women is generally defined as defending women's rights. But I believe that by doing so I am also defending men's rights. Women are the *prima facie* victims of violence and discrimination, but men are also victims. When you violate women's rights, restrict their development and treat them as second-class citizens, you create an unstable marital relationship and an unbalanced family. This takes its toll not only on women, but on husbands, children and the whole of society."[55]

The global aid agency Oxfam Great Britain, along with the Lebanese women's rights organization, KAFA, has released the first-ever pan-Arab training guide on practical ways to engage men and boys in the fight to end violence against women. The title of this guide is "Women and Men . . . Hand in Hand Against Violence." Oxfam GB and KAFA have been jointly running a pilot initiative in the Bekaa Valley region of Lebanon and hope to replicate the successful project in other Arab countries. Ghida Anani, KAFA program coordinator of the joint project, said: "Men are part of the problem, but they are also part of the solution. We are against violence, not men. But men in the Arab world almost always dominate the public and private spheres so working with them is strategically critical. If we want to begin making real change in ending violence against women it is simply nonsensical to leave men and boys out of the equation whether it's in Lebanon, Iraq, Egypt, Yemen or anywhere in the world for that matter." In its physical, psychological, and sexual forms, violence against women can be found in the household, the community, and public institutions. Furthermore, it has serious economic, social, and health implications for the whole family, including men and boys. Ghida Anani added: "Poverty increases violence, and in turn, violence increases poverty as abused women are often unable to help support the family. It undermines and destroys women's dignity, confidence, and self-respect, often preventing them from seeking out and taking advantage of opportunities that could better their lives and that of their families. While it is important that women learn about their own rights and how to receive help if they are abused, it is at least equally important that the mindset that allows for men to commit acts of violence begins to change. Because once that changes, the abuse itself will decline."[56]

In summary, the seven strategies that have been presented above have proven to be effective ways to undertake bottom-up changes that would benefit women by decreasing the wounds they receive, healing the wounds they have, and increasing their physical security, their equity in the family and

future aggression. Because violence is perpetuated only when it is viewed by the perpetrator as functional or effective in providing what it is that the perpetrator wants, systematically denying the reward or sought-after result will soon extinguish the behavior. It is important, however, that gender violence *never* be allowed to be functional. Even if violence is only occasionally functional, the tendency to be violent will be strengthened, because at each occurrence the perpetrator will gamble that this time will be the time when the desired reward will be forthcoming. It should be remembered that this is only the first step in improving conditions for women. Violence prevention simply helps men and women coexist without overt aggression by repressing violent and antisocial behaviors; it does not teach higher-order social skills that directly help develop peaceful relations between men and women, but it is a necessary step.

Because of the critical role that punishment plays in preventing violence, and the role that laws play in defining what behavior is to be acceptable and what behavior is to be punished, it is very important to keep track of proposed laws and the opinions of those who both oppose and support them. This process is especially important when both sides of the issue see their opinions as being in concert with the teachings of the broader culture. As we mentioned in chapter 2, in March 2009 Afghan legislators quietly passed a law that allows a husband to demand intercourse with his wife every four days. The law, which applies only to the Shi'a of Afghanistan, also determines when and why a wife can go out of her home alone. Appalled at Afghanistan's backsliding, more than a hundred protesters in Kabul called for the law to be repealed, saying it did nothing but legalize marital rape. They were challenged by more than eight hundred counter-protesters who vilified their opponents as agents of the West and not true to Islam. In an effort to defuse the issue, Afghan president Karzai—under intense Western pressure—suspended enforcement and remanded the law to the Justice Department for review. It would have been better if bottom-up forces in Afghan society had had in place a mechanism to monitor the development of such government initiatives, so that pressure, even if that pressure was foreign, could have been applied before the debate became public, since the public debate encouraged open demonstration of the lamentable view that protecting women was somehow un-Islamic.

Even when laws are passed, the challenges associated with implementing and enforcing them are enormous and require scrutiny and vigilance by bottom-up forces. Years after passing the much-hailed 2004 Moudawana (Family Code), which we outlined in chapter 5, Morocco is still struggling

in such cases and simultaneously publicized, sexual harassment would greatly decrease. As long as men think they can get away with it, they will continue to do it. A culture of male impunity must be replaced by a culture of strict male accountability.

Even when a behavior is not illegal, strategic publicizing of shocking events can change the political and social context, allowing new legislation to be passed criminalizing what was previously acceptable in society. In May 2009, after three formal attempts, an eight-year-old girl was finally granted a divorce from her fifty-year-old husband in Saudi Arabia.[61] The case reopened the debate about the propriety and legality of allowing young girls to marry. In response to the trial, Saudi columnist Amal al-Zahid called for the outlawing of the "trafficking of child brides—a most reactionary practice that takes us back to the days of concubines [and] slave girls." In a similar and more recent case in the same country, a twelve-year-old girl filed for a divorce from an eighty-year-old man—her father's cousin, whom she had been forced to marry a year earlier.[62] The government-run Human Rights Commission is providing a lawyer for the girl and activists are hoping that this case might result in establishing a minimum legal age for marriage. The government is clearly using the publicity surrounding these cases to press for reform. Once again, we see the pincer of top-down and bottom-up efforts working to produce a positive result. Saudi Arabia is now moving rapidly toward setting age sixteen as the minimum marriage age for girls.

Survivors who are willing to publicly recover from abuse and go on to live normal, happy lives provide another avenue to stymie the functionality of violence. As we mentioned earlier in the chapter, Mukhtar Mai was gang-raped by order of a village council as punishment for her brother's alleged illicit relations with a woman from a rival clan. Rather than commit suicide, as many rape victims are expected to do, brave Mukhtar decided to stand up against her attackers in court where the charge against her brother was found to be a cover-up for a different sex crime committed by other clan members. As an additional sign of bravery, Mukhtar then agreed to become the second wife of the policeman who was assigned to guard her when she pressed charges against the rapists. Once again, she shattered the taboos that generally relegate rape survivors to suicide or to a life with no hope of ever marrying. Through her use of legal and social processes to keep her rapists from covering up the real crime and also her determination against all odds to reclaim a normal, happy life, she has become "a symbol of hope for voiceless and oppressed women" in Pakistan.[63]

about how they should behave, which they have learned in the context of growing up in families from various traditions and cultures. As children express themselves within family life, their patterns of behavior are shaped by the consequences of their actions, experienced primarily through the reactions of others. Behavior that is successful in getting individuals the rewards they want will be repeated, while behavior that is not effective in obtaining the desired results will be less likely to appear again. In cultures where amicable male-female relationships have never been seen or reinforced, young people do not learn how to interact in mutually supportive ways with the other sex. They do not know how to avoid the possibility of gender conflict, and if such conflict occurs, they have no idea of how to resolve it without violence. Asking men and women to live together with respect and equity in such societies may be asking them to behave in ways that are utterly foreign to them. They simply do not know how to go about it.

Therefore, the next step in the fight against gender violence and exploitation is to provide scripts of interaction when they are absent in society. Researchers have found that new patterns of behavior can be created through the use of such scripts. These can prescribe what to say in the middle of tense moments or how to break down dysfunctional gender stereotypes and create new, healthy, respectful ones. Techniques used by the advertising industry to great effect, such as songs and jingles, can sometimes be used to help women and men remember what to do in given circumstances. Once memorized, they become guidelines of what to say in similar situations. Individuals can also create gender-appropriate behavior, and these examples can be used to posit new definitions of what it means to be a girl or a boy, a woman or a man. People can be encouraged to develop definitions that might portray men as considerate of their wives and daughters and dedicated to the development of their talents and abilities. Furthermore, it would be a great deterrent to violence against women if male stereotypes included the idea that men's self-esteem and eminence derive from positive, peaceful behavior toward women. The societal measure of a man, rather than the degree of domination and control over the women in his life, should be how well he appreciates them and to what extent he helps them become healthy and educated participants in all aspects of life.

Alexander B. Morrison, a religious authority with whom we are familiar, had the calling to travel and interact with members of his church in other lands. He found ways to inculcate a new definition of manhood through example. At a dinner attended by the local ecclesiastical authorities and their

who have prolonged urinary tract infections and kidney and liver problems because they don't have a safe place to go."

Previous attempts to bring toilets to poor Indian villages mostly failed. A 2001 project sponsored by the World Bank never took off because many people used the latrines as storage facilities or took them apart to build lean-tos. But linking toilets to courtship—"No Toilet, No Bride"—has been the most successful effort so far. Walls in many villages are painted with the slogan, and popular soap operas have featured dramatic plots involving the campaign. "The 'No Toilet, No Bride' program is a bloodless coup," said Bindeshwar Pathak, founder of Sulabh International, a social service organization and winner of the 2009 Stockholm Water Prize for developing inexpensive, eco-friendly toilets. "When I started, it was a cultural taboo to even talk about toilets. Now it's changing. My mother used to wake up at four a.m. to find someplace to go quietly. My wife wakes up at seven a.m. and can go safely in her home."

This mini-script that started with the toilets has resulted in other advantages as well. Pathak runs a school and job-training center for women who once cleaned up human waste by hand. They are known as untouchables, the lowest caste in India's social order. As more toilets come to India, women are less likely to have to do such jobs. "I want so much for them to have skills and dignity," Pathak said. These four little words, "No Toilet, No Bride," are also helping women to see themselves as having value, and to see that they are valuable enough that they deserve a toilet before they marry. Their potential husbands also begin to see the women as having more value, as someone for whom they may have to obtain the required toilet. The jingle also gives a woman something to say if a young suitor does not provide her with a toilet—she has a socially approved script to follow, and society will justify her decision to refuse the marriage.[65]

Drama has always been a pivot point for massive social change, and some television programs have been helpful to both women and men by demonstrating new ways for them to interact. The powerful influence of television is noted by Iranian feminist Syma Sayah, who states: "Satellite has shown an alternative way of being. Women see that it is possible to be treated equally with men."[66] One of the more noted shows that models new gender interaction behavior is the Turkish soap opera *Noor*. After being dubbed into colloquial Syrian Arabic, this show became an instant hit in the Arab world. Dubbed foreign soap operas are nothing new to the region, but what is new

quota. I call that a total revolution." A few years later the proportion of women in the parliament was increased to 12 percent and Hagi was elected as one of its members.[69] None of this would have happened if Hagi had not been able to write a new political script that included a new Sixth Clan representing more than half of the people of Somalia—the women.

Patterns for behaving in a more respectful and healing manner can also be instantiated in new rituals that can be adopted by the society. Even more tragic than African girls being abducted to fight in rebel forces is that when they are able to return to their communities, they are rejected. It is a very long and difficult process for them, inasmuch as they do not receive the same assistance boys receive to help them become reintegrated into the society. Furthermore, girls who have violated cultural gender norms through aggressive behavior and being raped experience enormous shame and guilt. Families and communities, unprepared or unwilling to accept them, often harass, threaten, and sexually or physically abuse them, leaving them with little hope that they will be able to work or marry.

One effective way to heal and reconnect the girls to their communities in northern Uganda and Sierra Leone has been the use of new, community-created rituals. These prescribed rituals, coupled with religious prayers, songs, and dancing, symbolically sever the past from a future of reconciliation and forgiveness, a process that involves the aid of ancestors, wards off evil influences, and facilitates social reintegration. The rituals are varied, and some call for costly materials. For example, the reunion of one girl named Ann was marked by her stepping on an egg before entering the community, the sacrifice of a goat, and the community assembling to celebrate. Then, at the church, the members fasted, gave thanks to God, and allowed Ann to return to schooling. Even after long separations and manifold offenses, the instrument of these rituals has proven to be a highly effective scripted intervention in forgiving and forgetting, allowing for full reconciliation for these women, who otherwise would not receive it in the same way as their male counterparts do.[70]

Rituals have also been used as substitutes for more harmful practices. In Kenya some groups have created new rites of passage for girls that take the place of female circumcision in pronouncing a girl to have crossed into womanhood. Another possibility is to use rituals to celebrate in a woman's life what was formerly not recognized as an occasion for celebration, thereby adding value to the everyday lives of women and girls. In several Western societies, for example, families are now celebrating the first menstruation of

both male and female, constructive gender interactions will begin to appear. It is important to remember that peaceful relationships will not be created by just one thoughtful act; what is required will be continued explaining and reinforcing behavior that models equality among men and women. Eventually more peaceful behavior will begin to appear and will permeate social and political structures.[72]

As one parent discovered, gender equality can be taught:

We do not live in a complete bubble, but the outside world is somewhat limited because we do not watch TV. But that is not the only place where templates are given to our children. There have been two shockers for us in the last few months. Savannah, our middle child, mentioned that she would like to be a doctor (of course that changes several times a day between dancer, artist, teacher, mom, doctor etc). Conner, her older brother, abruptly told that she could not be a doctor. My wife and I made very clear that he was wrong and he even knew female doctors and that he had no right to try and limit his sister's dreams. On another occasion, Savannah was talking about girls in the army. Conner told her that girls could not be in the military because they were not strong enough. This time Savannah stood up to him and told him girls were strong! We watched them banter back and forth a little and then more gently this time told Conner that Savannah was correct, girls could be in the military. This was a little puzzling still to him, but he accepted it.

We weren't sure he had "gotten it," but then saw this teaching pay off at the bus stop later on. At the bus stop near our house, the elementary school boys have always enforced the rule that boys get on the bus first, and girls are last. On this particular day, we noticed that Conner was first in line, with his sister second. The other boys were trying to push her out of the way. Conner then intervened and insisted that Savannah, even though she was a girl, should not have to give up her place in line—and he held his ground as the other boys tried to get past him. That is when we knew that what we were teaching in the home was not falling on deaf ears, and that we had an obligation to teach our children what was right concerning how to treat the other sex.[73]

A change of perspective is not only for the young; it is also for the fully mature. In Japan, after a law was passed in 2003 giving a wife who files for divorce the right to claim up to half her husband's company pension, men

In his best-selling book, *Three Cups of Tea*, Greg Mortenson tells the story of Haji Ali, the village chief of Korphe in northern Pakistan, who sought Mortenson's help in building a school for the children of his village. When the school was almost completed, Haji Mehdi, a neighboring village chief who through intimidation and threats controlled the economy of the valley, came to Korphe to log his protest against the school and especially the schooling of girls—which he said was forbidden by Allah. When Haji Ali defended the school, Mehdi demanded that a price—twelve of the best rams from the village—be paid to ensure that the school would remain. Without hesitation, Haji Ali called for the rams, paid the bribe, and sent his neighbor and his henchmen on their way. Of that moment Mortenson writes: "Haji Ali had just handed over half the wealth of the village to that crook, but he was smiling like he had just won the lottery." Ali then assured the villagers that even though they had lost the rams, and even though Haji Mehdi would have food for that day, the children of Korphe would have 'education forever.'"[76]

When gender equality has been internalized, even searing introspection and great sacrifice in its pursuit become deeply meaningful. When the heart has changed, it takes no effort to change one's actions; they spring forth from us without necessity of coercion. True, lasting, powerful change comes only with the internalization of a healthy understanding of who women really are, and why they are worth changing for.

WHAT CAN YOU PERSONALLY DO TO REDUCE VIOLENCE AGAINST WOMEN AND FURTHER PEACE?

You have the opportunity to join the most important movement of the twenty-first century—the movement to reduce violence against women and in that way to help establish household, local, national, and even international peace. In addition to joining the existing organized efforts that are under way in every nation today, as this chapter has detailed, internalization of gender equity must start with a moral inspection of our own everyday lives. The following benchmarks might be helpful to you in this important endeavor.

REFUSE TO PARTICIPATE IN ANY ACTIVITY THAT MIGHT TRAIN YOU TO PERPETUATE GENDER VIOLENCE

For Xhosa women in South Africa, marriage may involve physical and psychological abuse. Many wondered how such norms were perpetuated. Know-on an evening out or considering acts of physical intimacy, the decision as to where and how far you go with a member of the other sex must be mutually decided upon. No intimidation or manipulation should ever be used to get your way, by either gender. This includes not only physical coercion but also psychological coercion. No woman should ever have to feel she "owes" anyone anything if that person is nice to her. No person, male or female, should feel used in a relationship.

A rising problem in the United States is the effect of pornography on respectful gender relationships. We have seen evidence that girls are repeatedly lied to and manipulated into relationships, even marriage, by young men who have secret addictions to pornography. The insidious impact of this addiction begins to be apparent when the new husband or boyfriend starts to criticize and then ridicule the woman's body. The verbal attacks are usually more than demeaning—they are psychologically abusive and destroy the self-confidence of the young woman, blaming her for the man's own problems and asking her to participate in degrading sexual activities. As the true nature of the young man's addiction to pornography becomes clear, the damage to the shattered young woman may be irreversible. Such instances of relationship fraud are becoming common fare in many countries throughout the world. If a young man who claims to love a young woman can put her through such torture, is it any wonder that he becomes capable of condoning collective violence against women or even other groups?

It is not only in relationships with intimate others that our allegiance to gender equality, or our betrayal of it, may be seen. How do we treat our mothers, our sisters, our daughters, our female colleagues? Do we actually hear what the women in our lives speak to us about? Do we dismiss their authority to speak on any specific topic because they are women? Do we think of them only as instrumentalities to fulfill our needs, or do we view them as whole human beings with independent wills and perspectives and needs of their own? Do we feel that no decision would be a sound one without asking for their views? Or do we believe that men have the final say on important decisions regardless of the position of women? Do we put women in impossible double binds, such as encouraging them to speak, but then considering them bossy if they do speak? Or believing that a woman can be nice or competent at what she does, but not both? Do we address accomplished women by their first names but address accomplished men by their titles?

One of our male students recounted an anecdote that has stayed with us. He was attending a reunion of people, men and women, who had worked

capable of retrieving what he himself forgot. I then proceeded to give them this explanation:

The use of the term "woman" was the point of the contention. In biological terms, the young man had correctly stated the sex of the young lady. However, by stating "woman" to the young lady, the young man wanted to parade his dominance in the relationship to all those present and especially to the young lady. He wanted to let her know that he was the dominant character in the relationship, thus his needs and wants came before hers. To many his behavior should be a clear warning sign of a relationship with future problems. It should never be necessary to show dominance in this type of relationship due to the simple fact that both needs and wants of both the man and woman are equal in importance and must be satisfied through cooperation and sacrifice. The use of dominating labels and titles between a man and woman in a relationship does nothing but degrade trust and cooperation.

The effects of such behavior are clearly shown by the young woman's reactions. First, she began to complete the task order by the young man, showing submission to his will. Secondly, and the more shocking of reactions to my mind, was the lack of support or voice from her when I corrected the young man. She sat there quietly, almost embarrassed that another had to step in [with] an act of prevention. During my explanation she laughed and giggled with him so as to show that she did not want to upset him by agreeing with me. The young woman showed clear signs of submission and lack of will. Sadly, many of the people who will read this know other women who are suffering in a submissive relationship. The question I pose is why women submit to this or choose to be in these types of relationships? As a young man, other men tell me to go to the gym and gain muscle because women love to feel safe and protected by a strong man, but yet many of these men feel the need to use this power not to protect but instead to dominate the woman in the relationship. I feel strongly that this is wrong and unhealthy, and I support the understanding that a relationship is a partnership of understanding and love towards one another's needs and wants to create harmony and trust, not domination. But the question remains, why do women submit?[78]

Clearly, enacting male domination and permitting male domination both need critical examination; as much introspection is needed by women as by men in order to erase the bad old ways of gender inequality.

contributions to her children, her family, and her nation. If every woman was in a relationship where there was no fear, but rather deep appreciation for her views and all of her contributions to the marriage and to the family, both men and women would flourish in the emotional security of true partnership. If the law reflected the same appreciation for female life and concerns as it does for male, the entire society would be based on equity and fairness, and a single standard of integrity would be applicable to all. Investing in women in fundamental ways, such as seeing that girls were educated to a level equal to that of boys, would ensure that nations were more likely to be prosperous, to be healthy, to be stable, and to be meaningfully democratic. If women were to make up a substantial percentage of corporate boards, their aversion to risky investments and corruption would likely diminish the number of banking failures and strengthen the global economy. If women were also consulted in decision making at all levels, the decisions would lead to better consequences overall, because they would have been made on the basis of the thoughtfulness of all the people, not just half of the people.

Imagine a world with double the intellectual and creative talent available to help solve unprecedented global problems such as escalating violence, economic crises, and global warming. Such problems demand that every available ounce of mind power and life experience be fully utilized in finding solutions. Women have the potential to play a key role in helping this world reach its next level of development, not by taking over the world but by standing shoulder to shoulder as equal partners with the men of their societies.

Removing obstacles to women's progress will also eliminate the detrimental effects on children now being raised by distressed mothers who are subjected to all kinds of injustices. Can you imagine what removing the suffering of these mothers would do to maximize the capabilities of their children—all the world's children? Fully functioning children would likely double again the creative forces available to alleviate crises in the world as well as eliminate some of the problems caused by troubled youth. The world has never witnessed the effects on generations of children who have been raised by self-actualized mothers. If your own mother had been free from the stresses of being female in a world grossly inequitable to females, how would your life be different? And would your peers' lives be different as well?

Finally, those societies that have greater levels of gender equality will be less likely to resort to conflict and warfare to secure their national interests. If the systemic insecurity of half of the world's population is reduced, the insecurity of the nations of the world will also be significantly diminished.

7

TAKING WING

The world of humanity is possessed of two wings: the male and the female. So long as these two wings are not equivalent in strength, the bird will not fly. Until womankind reaches the same degree as man, until she enjoys the same arena of activity, extraordinary attainment for humanity will not be realized; humanity cannot wing its way to heights of real attainment. When the two wings ... become equivalent in strength, enjoying the same prerogatives, the flight of man will be exceedingly lofty and extraordinary.[1]

THERE IS SOMETHING spectacular about watching a bird take flight: a flock of flamingos awkwardly rising from the water; a single kingfisher leaving its perch on an overhanging branch to drop down into the water to spear a fish; a robin returning with food to her nest of hungry babies. More often than not it is in the security and protection of trees that birds seek refuge and from which birds take flight.

That image of birds and the trees that harbor them echoes the theme of roots and wings that we have developed over the course of this book. Roots, no matter the depth or direction of growth, are crucial for the survival of the tree. When they are neglected, abused, or cut off, the tree suffers and perhaps even dies. Throughout history, the perspectives of women have likewise been ignored, their labor exploited and their rights curtailed. The outcome is a world out of balance; a world less secure, less humane, and less wise than it otherwise would be.

Likewise, when a bird's wing has been injured or broken through violence, the bird will not be able to fly. If the women have never had the opportunity to experience a true "peacetime" in their lives, the lives of not only women but also men and children will be crippled and unable to reach their full potential. Without healing for women, the world of states will continue to be unstable and insecure. Are we willing to let it all continue? Who would really benefit from such a continuation? We argue that the answer is no one: no one, male or female, old or young, benefits from the wounding of women.

7

TAKING WING

The world of humanity is possessed of two wings: the male and the female. So long as these two wings are not equivalent in strength, the bird will not fly. Until womankind reaches the same degree as man, until she enjoys the same arena of activity, extraordinary attainment for humanity will not be realized; humanity cannot wing its way to heights of real attainment. When the two wings . . . become equivalent in strength, enjoying the same prerogatives, the flight of man will be exceedingly lofty and extraordinary.[1]

THERE IS SOMETHING spectacular about watching a bird take flight: a flock of flamingos awkwardly rising from the water; a single kingfisher leaving its perch on an overhanging branch to drop down into the water to spear a fish; a robin returning with food to her nest of hungry babies. More often than not it is in the security and protection of trees that birds seek refuge and from which birds take flight.

That image of birds and the trees that harbor them echoes the theme of roots and wings that we have developed over the course of this book. Roots, no matter the depth or direction of growth, are crucial for the survival of the tree. When they are neglected, abused, or cut off, the tree suffers and perhaps even dies. Throughout history, the perspectives of women have likewise been ignored, their labor exploited and their rights curtailed. The outcome is a world out of balance; a world less secure, less humane, and less wise than it otherwise would be.

Likewise, when a bird's wing has been injured or broken through violence, the bird will not be able to fly. If the women have never had the opportunity to experience a true "peacetime" in their lives, the lives of not only women but also men and children will be crippled and unable to reach their full potential. Without healing for women, the world of states will continue to be unstable and insecure. Are we willing to let it all continue? Who would really benefit from such a continuation? We argue that the answer is no one: no one, male or female, old or young, benefits from the wounding of women.

constitutional reform committee created in Egypt had no women members; the draft of the revisions to the constitution indicated that only a man can stand for president in Egypt; the interim cabinet contained no women at all; and the quota for women in parliament was summarily eliminated. That this should be the case is unsurprising: men see men as the only other "real" players in the game of politics. When power issues become serious, attention to women's voices disappears while the men cut the cards among themselves and for themselves. Women's activists decided to demonstrate publicly to remind the men that they were there and wanted a place at the table, but only a few hundred women showed up—to face a crowd of anti-women protesters shouting slogans like "Men are men and women are women and that will never change and go home, that's where you belong,"[5] The *Christian Science Monitor* reported, "'Go home, go wash clothes,' yelled some of the men. 'You are not married; go find a husband.' Others said, 'This is against Islam.' To the men demonstrating with the women, they yelled, 'Shame on you!' Suddenly, the men decided the women had been there long enough. Yelling, they rushed aggressively upon the protest, pushing violently through the rows of women. The women scattered. Eyewitnesses said they saw three women being chased by the crowd. A surge of men followed them, and Army officers fired shots into the air to make the men retreat."[6]

Yes, this is the same Tahrir Square in which women and men stood side by side to gain their freedom just a few weeks before this spectacle. The *Monitor* quoted one Egyptian woman taking part in the march as saying, "'They can't just send us home after the revolution.'" Well, that is the issue, isn't it? Can "they"? And what would the United States and the international community be prepared to do to prevent that from happening?

As we discussed in chapter 5, now is the time for the international community—and the United States—to develop an R2PW action plan for situations such as what we see in Afghanistan and Egypt today. Instead of dropping women like irrelevant "pet rocks," we need to be thinking creatively about how the world can avoid regressing in the areas of women's rights. It is absolutely true that only Afghan women, Egyptian women, Tunisian women, and Yemeni women can protect their own rights. That is true for the women of every nation, even the United States. But they have always needed partners, public support, and material assistance.

The first step is to understand in the fullest sense possible that the security of states is in fact linked to the security of women—and that that is not the idealist position but the realist position. Those who adhere to the tenets of

Our own empirical research buttresses Bachelet's assertions. We have found in conventional aggregate empirical testing that the best predictor of a state's peacefulness is not its level of wealth, or its level of democracy, or whether it is Islamic or not. The very best predictor of a state's peacefulness is its level of violence against women. Even democracies with poor physical security for women are less peaceful than democracies with good physical security for women. The greater the inequity in family law concerning women, the less stable and the less peaceful the nation. And the less willing a country is to enforce laws protecting women within its own borders, the less likely it is to comply with international treaty obligations. These empirical findings, we believe, are only the tip of the iceberg. As we develop our database and make it more comprehensive and longitudinal in nature, we believe we will not only confirm these initial findings but expand them as well.

And ours are not the only findings that underscore the link between the security of women and the security of states. As we more fully outlined in chapter 4, scholars have found that the larger the gap between men and women in the society, the more likely a nation is to be involved in intra- and interstate conflict, to be the aggressor, to use force first in a conflict, and to resort to higher levels of violence in a conflict. And, of course, if one turns to issues of national health, economic growth, corruption, and social welfare, the best predictors are those that incorporate measures of the situation of women. The days when one could claim that the situation of women had nothing to do with matters of national or international security are, frankly, over. The empirical results to the contrary are just too numerous and too robust.

Acknowledgment of this reality, then, is the first, foundational step. The second step is for the international community to devote the resources necessary to develop a meaningful set of indicators on the situation of women that can be monitored and tracked over time. Regress for women can happen suddenly, it can happen surreptitiously, and it can happen under the radar of the large media outlets. For example, though it is illegal in Russia to require women to wear a headscarf, Chechnya has begun to force such a dress code on women. Women are prohibited from going to school or working for the government if they do not wear the headscarf. Men on the streets, egged on by Chechnya's provincial leader, have taken to shooting women with paintball guns if they are not wearing headscarves.[8] The Kremlin has not uttered one word of protest about these activities. If a monitoring system were in place, this issue would now be on the to-do lists of not only UN Women, not only

tary of State Hillary Clinton said she speaks about this issue when she is in contact with Egyptian officials: "Because it would be a shame, with all of the extraordinary change that's going on in Egypt if women were somehow not given their opportunity to be part of bringing about the new Egypt. . . . I think it's important that we always raise it, because we think it will be a better outcome. We don't want to see Egypt, or Tunisia, or any place eliminate half the population when they think about the future. That would make no sense at all."[9] Apparently her concerns have not caused the Egyptians, at least, to include any women in their transitional government: perhaps even when one is U.S. Secretary of State, some still believe a woman's voice can be ignored. We need male American officials at the highest level, including the president of the United States, to speak out both publicly and privately on this issue.

In Afghanistan, we need to be thinking in concrete terms about how to ensure a softer landing for Afghan women when American forces leave. Specific measures would include setting up the following legal and practical infrastructure before we leave: an asylum policy for Afghan women who face the threat of femicide; a scholarship program to take the best and brightest female Afghan students into U.S. universities; assurance that women are well represented in the peace *jirga* talks with the "moderate" Taliban; pursuing indictments in the International Criminal Court (ICC) against top Taliban leaders who have ordered femicide; complete funding for a Radio Free Women of Afghanistan station; establishing mosque-based female education, which locations would be less likely to be attacked; insisting to the Afghan government that women's shelters should not be taken over by the government; and finally, continuing to tie aid to Afghanistan to specific and measurable improvements in the situation of women in that land—including assisting them with the kinds of projects that protect female inheritance and land rights.

We are not helpless, either as individual nations or as the international community, when faced with a poor or worsening situation for women in the countries of the world. First, we need to nip retrogression in the bud through strong and united support of those in the affected country who oppose such retrogression; next, we need to assist women in countries where baseline conditions need improvement. We can do this.

Nearly a century ago, nations fought a war to end all wars. While noble in intent, that effort was a failure. Perhaps the world is now ready for another effort to ensure world peace. We are recommending one important and strategic front where that battle should be waged—in healing the wounds that

On the basis of the research we have laid out in this volume, we believe the primary challenge facing the twenty-first century is to eliminate violence against women and remove the barriers to the development of their strength and creativity and voice. Establishing gender equality in interpersonal relationships, in homes, in the workplace, and in decision-making bodies at all levels will change states and their behaviors, and in turn will bring prosperity and peace to the world. The three wounds—the physical insecurity of women, inequity in family law, and lack of parity in the councils of human decision making—must be attended to with all vigilance and care at levels both high and humble.

A bird with one broken wing will never soar. We know that; our species has experienced it for millennia, and paid for that sure knowledge with rivers of blood and mountains of needless suffering. The nations of the world must try a different path, a path that we have every reason to believe will lead to greater well-being, prosperity, security, and peace for the entire international system—the path of equality between men and women.

We cannot fail . . . it's time for the bird to finally take wing.

APPENDIX A

OPERATIONALIZATIONS FOR DATA ANALYSIS IN CHAPTER 4

To test the hypotheses listed in chapter 4, each variable must be operationalized.

- Physical Security of Women, operationalized as the Physical Security of Women (PSOW) scale. This five-point ordinal scale attempts to capture the degree of physical threat experienced by women generally within the society. The scale focuses in particular on the level of violence against women, including the prevalence of domestic violence, rape, marital rape, and murder of women in the nation. These subcomponents are examined in terms of custom, practice, law, and statistics related to these four forms of violence against women. This index is coded as MULTIVAR-SCALE-1 in the WomanStats Database; coded July 2007; coding scheme outlined in the codebook found at http://womanstats.org/CodebookCurrent.htm#psow.

- Physical Security of Women Index Including Son Preference (PSOWSP) scale. Using the ordinal PSOW score as a baseline, this variant includes the degree to which son preference is present within a society, and to what degree such a preference is enacted in society by offspring sex selection. That is, not only is the physical security of existing women important, but it is certainly a matter of physical security for women if the births of female fetuses are selectively precluded. The variable ISSA-SCALE-1 in the WomanStats Database is thus used to supplement the PSOW scale point for each nation; coded February 2007; coding scheme found in codebook listed above.

- Physical Security of Women Minus Marital Rape (PSOWMMR) scale. Because PSOW as normally scaled includes an examination of marital rape, which is also a variable examined by the Inequity in Family Law scale, we engaged in a recoding of the 2009 PSOW that eliminated marital rape as a con-

democracy, including the Polity IV data, the Freedom House measures are often used in international relations scholarship; they offer a methodological advantage in this particular analytic effort in that polytomous logistic regression results can be affected by a serious mismatch in number of scale points between independent and dependent variables. Our dependent variables are all five-point scales; Freedom House is a three-point scale, and Polity IV is a twenty-one-point scale. We used the Freedom House data coded 2007; www .freedomhouse.org/template.cfm?page=1.

- Level of Wealth, operationalized as GDP per capita. Although GDP per capita is a crude measure, it is often used in empirical analysis for its broad indication of level of national wealth and economic development. In our analysis, we use GDP per capita as coded by CIA World Factbook, 2007, countries identified by quintile; https://www.cia.gov/library/publications/the-world-factbook/index.html.

- Prevalence of Islamic Civilization. This scale indicates the degree to which adherence to the Islamic religion is prevalent within the nation. This dichotomous variable is coded by S. Matthew Stearmer and Chad F. Emmett in "The Great Divide: Revealing Differences in the Islamic World Regarding the Status of Women and Its Impact on International Peace" (paper presented at the annual meeting of the American Political Science Association, Chicago, August 29–September 1, 2007. http://womanstats.org/StearmerEmmettAPSA 07.pdf.

- Inequity in Family Law/Practice (IFL) scale. This scale was developed by Rose McDermott and was coded in 2007 (Rose McDermott, "MULTIVAR-SCALE-3," http://womanstats.org/CodebookCurrent.htm#inequity, 2007). The index utilizes the information provided by the WomanStats Database, the largest and most comprehensive database concerning the status of women in the world, coding for more than 320 variables in 175 countries (http://woman stats.org). McDermott chose to examine law and practice concerning age of marriage, polygyny, consent in marriage, abortion, divorce, whether marital rape is recognized as a crime, and inheritance law and practices. McDermott scales these variables along a five-point ordinal scale, ranging from 0 to 4, with the 0 scale point representing equitable family law/practice and 4 representing highly inequitable family law/practice. McDermott has placed the definitions of her scale points online (McDermott,2007), so we will not repeat those here; http://womanstats.org/CodebookCurrent.htm#inequity.

- Prevalence of Polygyny Scale. McDermott, originally coded in 2007 and then recoded according to new scale points in 2009 (McDermott 2009).

APPENDIX B

DATA ANALYSIS RESULTS FOR CHAPTER 4

TABLE B.1 Chi-Square Results: Physical Security of Women (PSOW, PSOWSP) and Measures of State Security (GPI, SOCIC, RN)

VARIABLES	CHI-SQUARE (LIKELIHOOD RATIO)	DF	SIGNIFICANCE $P<$
PSOW and GPI	41.212	12	.0001
$N = 105$	(47.077)		
PSOWSP and GPI	36.623	12	.0001
$N = 105$	(44.162)		
PSOW and SOCIC	88.122	12	.0001
$N = 140$	(88.050)		
PSOWSP and SOCIC	78.136	12	.0001
$N = 140$	(84.320)		
PSOW and RN	45.884	12	.0001
$N = 106$	(46.438)		
PSOWSP and RN	44.029	12	.0001
$N = 106$	(44.697)		

Note: PSOW = Physical Security of Women; PSOWSP = Physical Security of Women and Son Preference; GPI = Global Peace Index; SOCIC = States of Concern to the International Community; RN = Relations with Neighbors

TABLE B.3 Multivariate Polytomous Logistic Regression of GPI (Global Peace Index) on Four Independent Variables Parameter Estimates

	ESTIMATE	STD. ERROR	WALD	DF	SIG.	95% CONFIDENCE INTERVAL LOWER BOUND	UPPER BOUND
Threshold [GPI = 1]							
Most Peaceful	−5.488	1.068	26.409	1	.000	−7.582	−3.395
[GPI = 2]	−1.958	.892	4.811	1	.028	−3.707	−.208
[GPI = 3]	.828	.869	.907	1	.341	−.875	2.530
[GPI = 4]	2.890	1.077	7.200	1	.007	.779	5.001
Location [PSOW = 1]							
Most Secure	−2.499	1.059	5.570	1	.018	−4.574	−.424
[PSOW = 2]	−1.570	.774	4.113	1	.043	−3.087	−.053
[PSOW = 3]	−.446	.586	.579	1	.447	−1.595	.703
[PSOW = 4]	0[a]	.	.	0	.	.	.
[Democracy = 1] Free	−.973	.652	2.224	1	.136	−2.252	.306
[Democracy = 2]	−.693	.610	1.288	1	.256	−1.889	.504
[Democracy = 3]	0[a]	.	.	0	.	.	.
[Wealth = 1] Wealthiest	−2.067	.949	4.745	1	.029	−3.926	−.207
[Wealth = 2]	−.844	.860	.962	1	.327	−2.530	.842
[Wealth = 3]	.469	.828	.320	1	.571	−1.154	2.092
[Wealth = 4]	.523	.880	.353	1	.553	−1.202	2.247
[Wealth = 5]	0[a]	.	.	0	.	.	.
[Islamic = 0] Non-Islamic	−.140	.647	.047	1	.828	−1.409	1.128
[Islamic = 1]	0[a]	.	.	0	.	.	.

Link function: Logit.
Note: GPI = Global Peace Index; PSOW = Physical Security of Women; Democracy = Level of Democracy; Wealth = Level of Wealth; Islamic = Prevalence of Islamic Civilization
[a]This parameter is set to zero because it is redundant.

TABLE B.4 (*continued*)

SYMMETRIC MEASURES

		VALUE	ASYMP. STD. ERROR[a]	APPROX. T[b]	APPROX. SIG.
Ordinal by Ordinal	Kendall's tau-b	.332	.092	2.721	.007
	Kendall's tau-c	.269	.099	2.721	.007
	Gamma	.778	.127	2.721	.007
	Spearman Correlation	.354	.098	2.727	.009[c]
Interval by Interval	Pearson's *R*	.334	.094	2.552	.014[c]
N of Valid Cases		54			

Note: GPI = Global Peace Index; PSOW = Physical Security of Women
[a]Not assuming the null hypothesis
[b]Using the asymptotic standard error assuming the null hypothesis
[c]Based on normal approximation

TABLE B.5 Ordinal by Ordinal Measures of Association (same as above, but using SOCIC (State of Concern to the International Community) as dependent variable)

SYMMETRIC MEASURES

		VALUE	ASYMP. STD. ERROR[a]	APPROX. T[b]	APPROX. SIG.
Ordinal by Ordinal	Kendall's tau-b	.417	.079	3.760	.000
	Kendall's tau-c	.357	.095	3.760	.000
	Gamma	.917	.085	3.760	.000
	Spearman Correlation	.441	.083	3.842	.000[c]
Interval by Interval	Pearson's *R*	.375	.067	3.161	.002[c]
N of Valid Cases		63			

[a]Not assuming the null hypothesis
[b]Using the asymptotic standard error assuming the null hypothesis
[c]Based on normal approximation

TABLE B.7 Cross-tabulation of Polygyny with GPI (Global Peace Index)

			\multicolumn{6}{c}{GPI ROUNDED[a]}
			\multicolumn{6}{c}{POLYGYNY 2007, 0–4 RANGE}
			0	1	2	3	4	TOTAL
GPI	1	Count	10	1	0	0	0	11
		% within GPI	90.9	9.1	0	0	0	100.0
		% within Polygyny 2007, 0-4 range	16.9	12.5	0	0	0	10.5
		% of Total	9.5	1.0	0	0	0	10.5
	2	Count	25	1	9	4	2	41
		% within GPI	61.0	2.4	22.0	9.8	4.9	100.0
		% within Polygyny 2007, 0-4 range	42.4	12.5	42.9	40.0	28.6	39.0
		% of Total	23.8	1.0	8.6	3.8	1.9	39.0
	3	Count	20	3	9	5	4	41
		% within GPI	48.8	7.3	22.0	12.2	9.8	100.0
		% within Polygyny 2007, 0-4 range	33.9	37.5	42.9	50.0	57.1	39.0
		% of Total	19.0	2.9	8.6	4.8	3.8	39.0
	4	Count	4	2	2	1	1	10
		% within GPI	40.0	20.0	20.0	10.0	10.0	100.0
		% within Polygyny 2007, 0-4 range	6.8	25.0	9.5	10.0	14.3	9.5
		% of Total	3.8	1.9	1.9	1.0	1.0	9.5
	5	Count	0	1	1	0	0	2
		% within GPI	0	50.0	50.0	0	0	100.0
		% within Polygyny 2007, 0–4 range	0	12.5	4.8	0	0	1.9
		% of Total	0	1.0	1.0	0	0	1.9
	Total	Count	59	8	21	10	7	105
		% within GPI	56.2	7.6	20.0	9.5	6.7	100.0
		% within Polygyny 2007, 0-4 range	100.0	100.0	100.0	100.0	100.0	100.0
		% of Total	56.2	7.6	20.0	9.5	6.7	100.0

(*continued*)

TABLE B.9 Polygyny's Association with RN (Relations with Neighboring Countries)

			ASYMP. STD.		APPROX.
		VALUE	ERROR[a]	APPROX. T[b]	SIG.
Ordinal by Ordinal	Kendall's tau-b	.284	.070	4.038	.000
	Kendall's tau-c	.232	.057	4.038	.000
	Gamma	.419	.100	4.038	.000
	Spearman Correlation	.336	.083	3.641	.000[c]
Interval by Interval	Pearson's R	.272	.078	2.881	.005[c]
N of Valid Cases		106			

SYMMETRIC MEASURES

[a]Not assuming the null hypothesis
[b]Using the asymptotic standard error assuming the null hypothesis
[c]Based on normal approximation

TABLE B.10 Polygyny's Association with Level of Organized Conflict (Internal)

SYMMETRIC MEASURES

			ASYMP. STD.		APPROX.
		VALUE	ERROR[a]	APPROX. T[b]	SIG.
Ordinal by Ordinal	Kendall's tau-b	.333	.067	4.844	.000
	Kendall's tau-c	.289	.060	4.844	.000
	Gamma	.461	.087	4.844	.000
	Spearman Correlation	.392	.078	4.704	.000[c]
Interval by Interval	Pearson's R	.406	.076	4.905	.000[c]
N of Valid Cases		124			

[a]Not assuming the null hypothesis
[b]Using the asymptotic standard error assuming the null hypothesis
[c]Based on normal approximation

TABLE B.14 Multivariate Polytomous Regression: GPI on IFL, Democracy, Wealth, Islamic Civilization

			PARAMETER ESTIMATES				95% CONFIDENCE INTERVAL	
		ESTIMATE	STD. ERROR	WALD	DF	SIG.	LOWER BOUND	UPPER BOUND
Threshold	[GPI = 1] Most Peaceful	-6.890	1.269	29.468	1	.000	-9.378	-4.402
	[GPI = 2]	-3.102	1.075	8.324	1	.004	-5.210	-.995
	[GPI = 3]	-.245	1.006	.059	1	.808	-2.217	1.728
	[GPI = 4]	1.932	1.176	2.700	1	.100	-.373	4.236
Location	[IFL = 0] Most Equitable	-3.713	1.195	9.660	1	.002	-6.054	-1.371
	[IFL = 1]	-1.626	.953	2.911	1	.088	-3.494	.242
	[IFL = 2]	-1.082	.905	1.431	1	.232	-2.856	.691
	[IFL = 3]	-1.823	.878	4.316	1	.038	-3.543	-.103
	[IFL = 4]	0[a]	.	.	0	.	.	.
	[Democracy = 2]	-.626	.620	1.021	1	.312	-1.841	.588
	[Democracy = 3]	0[a]	.	.	0	.	.	.
	[Wealth = 1] Wealthiest	-2.067	1.042	3.935	1	.047	-4.109	-.025
	[Wealth = 2]	-1.024	.988	1.074	1	.300	-2.961	.913
	[Wealth = 3]	.300	.985	.093	1	.761	-1.631	2.232
	[Wealth = 4]	.895	.924	.938	1	.333	-.916	2.706
	[Wealth = 5]	0[a]	.	.	0	.	.	.
	[Islamic = 0] Non-Islamic	-.774	.574	1.819	1	.177	-1.898	.351
	[Islamic = 1]	0[a]	.	.	0	.	.	.

Link function: Logit.

Note: IFL = Inequity in Family Law/Practice; GPI = Global Peace Index; Democracy = Level of Democracy; Wealth = Level of Wealth; Islamic = Prevalence of Islamic Civilization

[a]This parameter is set to zero because it is redundant.

NOTES

1. ROOTS OF NATIONAL AND INTERNATIONAL RELATIONS

1. A small minority of people are neither biologically male nor biologically female; they are intersex. Other individuals may be transsexual. In these cases, the perception of sex, rather than sex itself, may determine the societal treatment of such people. In some cultures it is possible to change gender even if sex is unchanged; for example, in Albania an ancient code allows women in certain circumstances to proclaim themselves to be men and to live as men, even though their sex remains acknowledged as female.

2. Jan Jindy Pettman, *Worlding Women: A Feminist International Politics* (New York: Routledge, 1996).

3. "Christian Man Who Got 39 Lashes and One Year in Jail Is Free," *Arabic News*, August 6, 1997, www.arabicnews.com/ansub/Daily/Day/970806/1997080619 .html, accessed May 18, 2010.

4. To access these variables, go to http://womanstats.org. The WomanStats Database codes for more than 320 variables concerning the situation of women in 175 countries. Access is free.

5. V. Spike Peterson, "Security and Sovereign States: What Is at Stake in Taking Feminism Seriously?" in V. Spike Peterson, ed., *Gendered States: Feminist (Re)Visions of International Relations Theory*, 31–64 (Boulder, CO: Lynne Rienner Publishers, 1992).

6. "Purdah" refers to the practice of sequestering women in private quarters and generally not allowing their entry into public space. "Infibulation" refers to a form of female genital cutting that involves sewing the stumped ends of cut labia together to form a seal with a tiny hole over the vaginal opening.

7. Valerie M. Hudson and Andrea M. Den Boer, *Bare Branches: The Security Implications of Asia's Surplus Male Population* (Cambridge, MA: MIT Press, 2004).

18. CNN, "Child Rape Survivor Saves 'Virgin Myth' Victims," June 5, 2009, www .cnn.com/2009/LIVING/06/04/cnnheroes.betty.makoni/index.html, accessed May 18, 2010.

19. Kristof and WuDunn, *Half the Sky*.

20. Marilyn Waring, *Counting for Nothing: What Men Value and What Women Are Worth*, 2nd ed. (Toronto: University of Toronto Press, 2004).

21. UNECA, "A Background Paper on Engendering Budgetary Policies and Pro-cesses," 2001, www.uneca.org/acgd/Publications/en_0112_latigo.pdf, accessed May 18, 2010.

22. See, for example, http://salary.com, accessed May 18, 2010.

23. FAO, "Food Needs and Population," World Food Summit, 1996, www.fao.org/ docrep/x0262e/x0262e23.htm, accessed May 18, 2010.

24. Claudia von Werlhof, "Women's Work: The Blind Spot in the Critique of Po-litical Economy," in Maria Mies, ed., *Women: The Last Colony*, 13–26 (Atlantic Highlands, NJ: Zed Books, 1988).

25. Ann Crittenden, *The Price of Motherhood* (New York: Henry Holt, 2001).

2. WHAT IS THERE TO SEE, AND WHY AREN'T WE SEEING IT?

1. John Ward Anderson and Molly Moore, "Third World Women: A Lifetime of Oppression," *International Herald Tribune*, February 15, 1993.

2. For a video of Suzanne Mubarak explaining her position on female genital cutting and others issues, see www.youtube.com/watch?v=S1oOgySZNvM, ac-cessed May 18, 2010.

3. Maggie O'Kane, "The Mistake of Being Muslim," *Guardian Weekly*, March 28, 1993, 9.

4. As recounted in Stephen Lewis, "Nairobi Press Conference on Ending Sexual Violence in the Eastern Region of the DRC," September 13, 2007, http://216.95.229.16/news_item.cfm?news=1988&year=2007, accessed May 18, 2010.

5. Anna Quindlen, "Victim and Valkyrie," *New York Times*, March 16, 1994, www .nytimes.com/1994/03/16/opinion/public-private-victim-and-valkyrie.html?sc p=2&sq=quindlen%20victim%20valkyrie%201994&st=cse, accessed May 18, 2010.

6. Dexter Filkins, "Afghan Girls, Scarred by Acid, Defy Terror, Embracing School," *New York Times*, January 13, 2009, www.nytimes.com/2009/01/14/wo rld/asia/14kandahar.html?scp=4&sq=acid%20attacks&st=cse, accessed May 18, 2010.

7. Pam Belluck, "Women's Killers Are Very Often Their Partners, Study Finds," *New York Times*, March 31, 1997, www.nytimes.com/specials/women/warchive/ 970331_1651.html, accessed May 18, 2010.

23. Christopher Guilmoto, "Sex Ratio Imbalance in Asia: Trends, Consequences, and Policy Responses," UNFPA, 2007, www.unfpa.org/gender/docs/studies/summaries/regional_analysis.pdf, accessed November 1, 2007.

24. A wonderful overview of this topic is Freda Banda's "Project on a Mechanism to Address Laws That Discriminate Against Women," Office of the High Commissioner for Human Rights, March 6, 2008, www.ohchr.org/Documents/Pub lications/laws_that_discriminate_against_women.pdf, accessed May 18, 2010.

25. "Om Gad," in Nayra Atiya, *Khul Khaal: Five Egyptian Women Tell Their Stories*, 14–15 (Syracuse, NY: Syracuse University Press, 1982).

26. Mohammed Jamjoom, "Age 12 Girl—Child Bride of Forced Marriage—Dies in Painful Childbirth, Infant Also Perishes," CNN, September 14, 2009, http://edition.cnn.com/2009/HEALTH/09/14/yemen.childbirth.death/index.html?iref=mpstoryview, accessed May 31, 2010.

27. Martha Nussbaum, *Sex and Social Justice* (Oxford: Oxford University Press, 2000).

28. Aditi Bhaduri, "Muslims in India Design New Marriage Contract," *Womens ENews*, August 4, 2008, www.womensenews.org/story/the-world/080804/mus lims-india-design-new-marriage-contract, accessed May 18, 2010.

29. Ann Crittenden, *The Price of Motherhood* (New York: Henry Holt, 2001).

30. Mehranguiz Kar and Homa Hoodfar, "Women and Personal Status Law in Iran," *Middle East Report*, no. 198 (January–March 1996): 36–38.

31. Stephanie Sinclair and Barry Bearak, "The Bride Price," *New York Times Magazine*, July 9, 2006, www.nytimes.com/2006/07/09/magazine/09BRI.html, accessed May 18, 2010.

32. Farah Stockman, "Women Pay a Price in War on Afghan Drug Trade," *Boston Globe*, September 28, 2005, www.boston.com/news/world/middleeast/articles/2005/09/28/women_pay_a_price_in_war_on_afghan_drug_trade/, accessed May 18, 2010.

33. Elizabeth Rubin, "Women's Work," *New York Times Magazine*, October 9, 2005, www.nytimes.com/2005/10/09/magazine/09afghan.html?pagewanted=1, accessed May 18, 2010.

34. Tabibul Islam, "Bangladesh: Rape Victims Married Off to Rapists," IPSNews, June16, 2003, http://ipsnews.net/interna.asp?idnews=18765, accessed May 18, 2010.

35. Calvin Sims, "Justice in Peru: Victim Gets Rapist for a Husband," *New York Times*, March 12, 1997, www.nytimes.com/1997/03/12/world/justice-in-peru-victim-gets-rapist-for-a-husband.html, accessed May 18, 2010.

36. Craig Smith, "Abduction, Often Violent, a Kyrgyz Wedding Rite," *New York Times*, April 30, 2005, www.nytimes.com/2005/04/30/international/asia/30brides.html, accessed May 18, 2010.

37. UNFPA, "Bride Kidnapping," 2006, www.unfpa.org/16days/documents/pl_bridenapping_factsheet.doc, accessed May 18, 2010.

women's-property-rights-takes-centre-stage-in-the-kenyan-media/, accessed May 18, 2010.

51. UNIFEM, "Women's Land and Property Rights," n.d., www.unifem.org/gender_issues/women_poverty_economics/land_property_rights.php, accessed May 18, 2010.

52. Certain female rulers, such as Queen Elizabeth I, were accorded male status and thus were not perceived as undermining the template.

53. Female leaders may be accorded male status as stand-ins for famous male relatives; here we think of Benazir Bhutto, Corazon Aquino, Violetta Chamorro, and others.

54. www.freerepublic.com/focus/news/811070/posts, accessed May 18, 2010.

55. www.freerepublic.com/focus/news/810823/posts, accessed May 18, 2010.

56. Washington Memorial Chapel, Valley Forge, Pennsylvania, http://209.200.101.38/?t=c&cid=13, accessed May 18, 2010. There is (finally) a movement in the United States to create a national monument dedicated to women who died as a result of pregnancy and childbirth; http://mothersmonument.org.

57. Quoted in Urvashi Butalia, "Mother India," OneWorld, March 7, 2001, www.oneworld.org/issue277/mother.htm, accessed May 18, 2010.

58. Arthur Gilbert and James Cole, "Revolutionary Theory and Gender Theory: The Iranian Case" (paper presented at the annual meeting of the International Studies Association, Chicago, February 21–25, 2005).

59. Harriet M. Johnston-Wood, "Letter to the Editor," New York Times, March 17, 1910, http://query.nytimes.com/mem/archive-free/pdf?res=9D0DE0DA1430E2 33A25752C2A9659C946196D6CF, accessed May 18, 2010.

60. Carol Cohn, "Wars, Wimps, and Women: Talking Gender and Thinking War," in Miriam Cooke and Angela Woollacott, eds., Gendering War Talk (Princeton, NJ: Princeton University Press, 1993), 227.

61. Inter-Parliamentary Union, "Women in National Parliaments," www.ipu.org/wmn-e/world.htm, accessed September 30, 2009.

62. Global Database of Quotas for Women, www.quotaproject.org/country.cfm, accessed May 18, 2010.

63. D. Kaufmann, "Challenges in the Next Stage of Corruption," in New Perspectives in Combating Corruption (Washington, D.C: Transparency International and the World Bank, 1998).

64. World Bank, "Engendering Development: Through Gender Equality in Rights, Resources, and Voice," World Bank Policy Research Report (Washington, DC: Oxford University Press, 2001).

65. Inter-Parliamentary Union, "Politics: Women's Insight," 2000, www.ipu.org/iss-e/women.htm, accessed December 26, 2007.

66. Ann Crittenden, If You've Raised Kids, You Can Manage Anything: Leadership Begins at Home (New York: Gotham, 2004), 76–77.

82. Some of the paragraphs that follow this sentence are adapted with permission from Valerie M. Hudson, "Good Riddance: Why Macho Had to Go," *Foreign Policy* (July/August 2009), www.foreignpolicy.com/articles/2009/06/19/good_riddance, accessed May 31, 2010.

83. Quoted in Michael Lewis, "Wall Street on the Tundra," *Vanity Fair*, April 2009, www.vanityfair.com/politics/features/2009/04/iceland200904, accessed May 18, 2010.

84. Brad Barber and Terrence Odean, "Boys Will Be Boys: Gender, Overconfidence, and Common Stock Investment," *Quarterly Journal of Investment* (February 2001): 261–291, http://faculty.haas.berkeley.edu/odean/papers/gender/BoysWillBeBoys.pdf, accessed May 18, 2010; Angela Lyons, Urvi Neelakantan, and Erik Scherpf, "Gender and Marital Differences in Wealth and Investment Decisions" (Networks Financial Institute Working Paper No. 2008-WP-02, 2008), http://papers.ssrn.com/sol3/papers.cfm?abstract_id=1109103, accessed May 18, 2010.

85. Chris Karpowitz and Tali Mendenberg, "Groups and Deliberations," *Swiss Political Science Review* 13, no. 4 (2007): 645–663; Chris Karpowitz and Tali Mendenberg, "Groups, Norms, and Gender: Initial Results from the Deliberative Justice Experiment" (paper presented at Southern California Political Psychology Workshop, University of California-Irvine, May 16, 2009).

86. Karpowitz and Mendenberg, "Groups, Norms, and Gender."

87. Marilyn Waring, *Counting for Nothing: What Men Value and What Women Are Worth*, 2nd ed. (Toronto: University of Toronto Press, 2004), 13.

88. UNDP, *The Human Development Report* (Oxford: Oxford University Press, 1995).

89. Salary.com, 9th Annual Mom Salary Survey, 2009, www.marketwire.com/press-release/SalaryCom-NASDAQ-SLRY-984585.html; Jennifer Steinhauer, "The Economic Unit Called Supermom," *New York Times*, May 8, 2005, 14, www.nytimes.com/2005/05/08/weekinreview/08stein.html?scp=1&sq=Steinhauer%202005%20supermom&st=cse, accessed May 18, 2010.

90. Crittenden, *The Price of Motherhood*.

91. Ibid.

92. Waring, *Counting for Nothing*, 3.

93. Nancy Folbre, *The Invisible Heart* (New York: New Press, 2001).

94. Waring, *Counting for Nothing*, 21, 10, 23, 65.

95. Harris Collingwood, "The Sink or Swim Economy," *New York Times Magazine*, June 8, 2003, www.nytimes.com/2003/06/08/magazine/the-sink-or-swim-economy.html?scp=2&sq=wet%20dreams%20economists&st=cse&pagewanted=4, accessed May 18, 2010.

96. Joan S. Williams, *Unbending Gender: Why Family and Work Conflict and What to Do About It* (Oxford: Oxford University Press, 2001).

6. United Nations Development Programme, "Arab Human Development Report 2005," http://hdr.undp.org/en/reports/regionalreports/arabstates/RBAS_ahdr 2005_EN.pdf, accessed May 31, 2010.

7. Bradley Thayer, *Darwin and International Relations: On the Evolutionary Origins of War and Ethnic Conflict* (Lexington: University Press of Kentucky, 2004), 8–9.

8. Richard Dawkins, *The Selfish Gene* (Oxford: Oxford University Press, 1989), 331.

9. Theodore D. Kemper, *Social Structure and Testosterone* (New Brunswick, NJ: Rutgers University Press, 1990), 138.

10. Richard D. Alexander, "Evolution and Culture," in Napoleon A. Chagnon and William Irons, eds., *Evolutionary Biology and Human Social Behavior: An Anthropological Perspective* (North Scituate, MA: Duxbury, 1979), 59–78, quote from 77.

11. Richard Wrangham and Dale Peterson, *Demonic Males: Apes and the Origins of Human Violence* (New York: Houghton Mifflin, 1996), 24–25.

12. Ibid., 231.

13. Barbara Smuts, "Male Aggression Against Women: An Evolutionary Perspective," *Human Nature* 3, no. 1 (1992): 1–44; Barbara Smuts, "The Evolutionary Origins of Patriarchy," *Human Nature* 6, no. 1 (1995): 1–32.

14. Smuts, "Evolutionary Origins of Patriarchy," p. 1.

15. When one turns to evolutionary theory's account of male-female relations formative evolutionary environment (FEE) of tens of thousands of years, one quickly finds two apparently contradictory viewpoints in the theoretical literature. One major school of thought, exemplified by the work of Wrangham and Peterson (*Demonic Males*), suggests that the FEE produced a generalized social system of male dominance hierarchies, encoding a deep hierarchical relationship between men and women whose long duration surely and profoundly shaped natural selection. However, another school of thought, exemplified by the work of Leacock (Eleanor Leacock, "Interpreting the Origins of Sexual Inequality: Conceptual and Historical Problems," *Dialectical Anthropology* 7 [1983]: 263–284), suggests that in the hunter-gatherer societies representative of the FEE, there was no generalized male dominance over females, and thus human beings and the collectives they form have not been subject to more than ten millennia of male dominance. Both schools concur that once agriculture and animal husbandry became mainstays of human food systems, approximately 10,000 years ago, generalized male dominance did arise globally across human societies. Maria Mies, "Social Origins of the Sexual Division of Labor," in Maria Mies, Veronika Bennholdt-Thomsen, and Claudia Von Werlhof, eds., *Women: The Last Colony*, 67–95 (London: Zed Books, 1988).

culture 10,000 years ago when women began to be confined to smaller spaces of home and land, and men, who became the suppliers of food and other resources, were able to exercise greater control over women and achieve parental certainty ("Sex Differences in Direct Aggression"). While male dominance hierarchies may have become entrenched at this time, male aggression and patriarchal practices are believed to have been one of the dominant strategies used in sexual selection during hunter-gatherer periods of human history (Smuts, "Evolutionary Origins of Patriarchy").

27. Smuts, "Evolutionary Origins of Patriarchy," 13, and Smuts, "Male Aggression Against Women," 15.

28. Napoleon A. Chagnon, "Life Histories, Blood Revenge, and Warfare in a Tribal Population," *Science* 239, no. 4843 (1988): 985–992.

29. Wrangham and Peterson, *Demonic Males*, 173.

30. Smuts, "Male Aggression Against Women," 11.

31. Ibid., 19.

32. Margo Wilson, Martin Daly, and Joanna Scheib, "Femicide: An Evolutionary Psychological Perspective," in Patricia Adair Gowaty, ed., *Feminism and Evolutionary Biology: Boundaries, Intersections, and Frontiers*, 431–465 (New York: Chapman and Hall, 1997).

33. Smuts, "Evolutionary Origins of Patriarchy," 18.

34. N. Pound, Martin Daly, and Margo Wilson, "There's No Contest: Human Sex Differences Are Sexually Selected," *Behavioral and Brain Sciences* 32, nos. 3/4 (2009): 286–287, quote from 286.

35. Mies, "Social Origins of the Sexual Division of Labor."

36. Smuts, "Evolutionary Origins of Patriarchy."

37. Smuts, "Male Aggression Against Women."

38. Ibid., 26.

39. Ibid., 6.

40. Smuts, "Evolutionary Origins of Patriarchy," 22.

41. Patricia Adair Gowaty, "Introduction: Darwinian Feminists and Feminist Evolutionist," in Patricia Adair Gowaty, ed., *Feminism and Evolutionary Biology: Boundaries, Intersections, and Frontiers*, 12 (New York: Chapman and Hall, 1997).

42. Wrangham and Peterson, *Demonic Males*, 125.

43. Ibid., 159.

44. Ibid., 146.

45. Barbara D. Miller, "The Anthropology of Sex and Gender Hierarchies," in Barbara D. Miller, ed., *Sex and Gender Hierarchies*, 22 (Cambridge: Cambridge University Press, 1993).

46. Kemper, *Social Structure and Testosterone*.

66. Cheryl Brown Travis, "Theory and Data on Rape and Evolution," in Cheryl Brown Travis, ed., *Evolution, Gender, and Rape*, 207–220 (Cambridge, MA: MIT Press, 2003).

67. Jacquelyn W. White and Lori A. Post, "Understanding Rape: A Metatheoretical Framework," in Cheryl Brown Travis, ed., *Evolution, Gender, and Rape*, 383–411 (Cambridge, MA: MIT Press, 2003).

68. John Archer, "Sex Differences in Aggression Between Heterosexual Partners: A Meta-analytic Review," *Psychological Bulletin* 126, no. 5 (2000): 651–680, doi: 10.1037/0033–2909.126.5.651.

69. John Archer, "Sex Differences in Aggression in Real-World Settings: A Meta-analytic Review," *Review of General Psychology* 8, no. 4 (2004): 291–322, doi: 10.1037/1089–2680.8.4.291.

70. Alice H. Eagly and Wendy Wood, "The Origins of Sex Differences in Human Behavior: Evolved Dispositions Versus Social Roles," *American Psychologist* 54, no. 6 (1999): 408–423.

71. Ibid., 421.

72. Wendy Wood and Alice H. Eagly, "A Cross-Cultural Analysis of the Behavior of Women and Men: Implications for the Origins of Sex Differences," *Psychological Bulletin* 128, no. 5 (2002): 699–727.

73. Ibid., 718.

74. Ibid., 722.

75. Stephanie H. M. van Goozen, Graeme Fairchild, and Gordon T. Harold, "The Role of Neurobiological Deficits in Childhood Antisocial Behavior," *Current Directions in Psychological Science* 17, no. 3 (2008): 224–228.

76. Adrian Raine, "Biosocial Studies of Antisocial and Violent Behavior in Children and Adults: A Review," *Journal of Abnormal Child Psychology* 30, no. 4 (2002): 311–325, www-rcf.usc.edu/~raine/BioSocialStudies_Raine.pdf, accessed May 31, 2010; Angela Scarpa and Adrian Raine, "Biosocial Bases of Violence," in Daniel J. Flannery, Alexander T. Vazsonyi, and Irwin D. Waldman, eds., *The Cambridge Handbook of Violent Behavior and Aggression*, 151–169 (Cambridge: Cambridge University Press, 2007).

77. Michael Bohman, "Predisposition to Criminality: Swedish Adoption Studies in Retrospect," in Gregory R. Bock and Jamie A. Goode, eds., *Genetics of Criminal and Antisocial Behavior*, 99–114 (West Sussex, UK: John Wiley, 1996); Remi J. Cadoret, Leslie D. Leve, and Eric Devor, "Genetics of Aggressive and Violent Behavior," *Anger, Aggression, and Violence* 20, no. 2 (1997): 301–322; Remi J. Cadoret, Colleen A. Cain, and R. R. Crowe, "Evidence for Gene-Environment Interaction in the Development of Adolescent Antisocial Behavior," *Behavior Genetics* 13 (1983): 301–310; Xiaojia Ge, Rand D. Conger, Remi J. Cadoret, Jenae M. Neiderhiser, William Yates, Edward Troughton, and Mark

88. M. Katherine Weinberg, Edward Z. Tronick, Jeffrey F. Cohn, and Karen L. Olson, "Gender Differences in Emotional Expressivity and Self-Regulation During Early Infancy," *Developmental Psychology* 35, no. 1 (1999): 175–188.

89. Patterson, "Comparison of Models."

90. Carol Lyon Martin, "A Ratio Measure of Gender Stereotyping," *Journal of Personality and Social Psychology* 52, no. 3 (1987): 489–499; Gerald R. Patterson, "Siblings: Fellow Travelers in Coercive Family Processes," *Advances in the Study of Aggression* 1 (1984): 173–214; Daniel S. Shaw and Emily Winslow, "Precursors and Correlates of Antisocial Behavior from Infancy to Preschool," in David M. Stoff, James Breiling, and Jack D. Maser, eds., *Handbook of Antisocial Behavior*, 148–158 (New York: John Wiley, 1997).

91. John D. Coie and Janis B. Kupersmidt, "A Behavioral Analysis of Emerging Social Status in Boy's Groups," *Child Development* 54 (1983): 1400–1416; Patterson, "Comparison of Models."

92. Brad J. Bushman and Russell G. Geen, "Role of Cognitive-Emotional Mediators and Individual Differences in the Effects of Media Violence on Aggression," *Journal of Personality and Social Psychology* 58, no. 1 (1990): 156–163; Nicholas L. Carnagey and Craig A. Anderson, "The Effects of Reward and Punishment in Violent Video Games on Aggressive Affect, Cognition, and Behavior," *Psychological Science* 16, no. 11 (2005): 882–889; Kenneth A. Dodge and Gregory S. Pettit, "A Biopsychosocial Model of the Development of Chronic Conduct Problems in Adolescence," *Developmental Psychology* 39, no. 2 (2003): 349–371; David P. Farrington, "Origins of Violent Behavior Over the Life Span," in Daniel J. Flannery, Alexander T. Vazsonyi, and Irwin D. Waldman, eds., *The Cambridge Handbook of Violent Behavior and Aggression*, 664–687 (Cambridge: Cambridge University Press, 2007); Holly Foster, Jeanne Brooks-Gunn, and Anne Martin, "Poverty/Socioeconomic Status and Exposure to Violence in the Lives of Children and Adolescents," in Daniel J. Flannery, Alexander T. Vazsonyi, and Irwin D. Waldman, eds., *The Cambridge Handbook of Violent Behavior and Aggression*, 664–687 (Cambridge: Cambridge University Press, 2007); Uberto Gatti, Richard E. Tremblay, and Frank Vitaro, "Iatrogenic Effect of Juvenile Justice," *Journal of Child Psychology and Psychiatry* 50, no. 8 (2009): 991–998, doi: 10.1111/j.1469–7610.2008 .02057.x; L. Rowell Huesmann and Lucyna Kirwil, "Why Observing Violence Increases the Risk of Violent Behavior by the Observer," in Daniel J. Flannery, Alexander T. Vazsonyi, and Irwin D. Waldman, eds., *The Cambridge Handbook of Violent Behavior and Aggression*, 545–570 (Cambridge: Cambridge University Press, 2007).

93. Elizabeth Reed, Jay G. Silverman, Anita Raj, Emily F. Rothman, Michele R. Decker, Barbara Gottlieb, Brett E. Mollar, and Elizabeth Miller, "Social and

107. E. Mark Cummings, Marcie C. Goeke-Morey, and Lauren M. Papp, "Every-day Marital Conflict and Child Aggression," *Journal of Abnormal Child Psychology* 32, no. 2 (2004): 191–202; Jeffrey L. Edleson, "Children's Witnessing of Adult Domestic Violence," *Journal of Interpersonal Violence* 14, no. 8 (1999): 839–870; Sandra A. Graham-Bermann, "The Impact of Woman Abuse on Children's Social Development: Research and Theoretical Perspectives," in George W. Holden and Robert Geffner, eds., *Children Exposed to Marital Violence: Theory, Research, and Applied Issues*, 21–54 (Washington, DC: American Psychological Association, 1998); Gayla Margolin and Elana B. Gordis, "The Effects of Family and Community Violence on Children," *Annual Review of Psychology* 51 (2000): 445–479.

108. Joetta L. Carr and Karen M. VanDeusen, "The Relationship Between Family of Origin Violence and Dating Violence in College Men," *Journal of Interpersonal Violence* 17, no. 6 (2002): 630–646, doi: 10.1177/0886260502017006003; Daniel J. Flannery, Mark I. Singer, Manfred van Dulmen, Jeff M. Kretschmar, and Lara M. Belliston, "Exposure to Violence, Mental Health, and Violent Behavior," in Daniel J. Flannery, Alexander T. Vazsonyi, and Irwin D. Waldman, eds., *The Cambridge Handbook of Violent Behavior and Aggression*, 306–321 (Cambridge: Cambridge University Press, 2007); Todd Herrenkohl, W. Alex Mason, Rick Kosterman, Liliana J. Lengua, J. David Hawkins, and Roberta D. Abbott, "Pathways from Physical Childhood Abuse to Partner Violence in Young Adulthood," *Violence and Victims* 19, no. 2 (2004): 123–136; M. Kay Jankowski, Harold Leitenberg, Kris Henning, and Patricia Coffey, "Intergenerational Transmission of Dating Aggression as a Function of Witnessing Only Same Sex Parents vs. Opposite Sex Parents vs. Both Parents as Perpetrators of Domestic Violence," *Journal of Family Violence* 14, no. 3 (1999): 267–279.

109. Bonnie Ballif-Spanvill, Claudia J. Clayton, and Suzanne B. Hendrix, "Witness and Nonwitness Children's Violent and Peaceful Behavior in Different Types of Simulated Conflict with Peers," *American Journal of Orthopsychiatry* 77, no. 2 (2007): 206–215.

110. Richard A. Fabes, Carol L. Martin, and Laura D. Hanish, "Young Children's Play Qualities in the Same-Other and Mixed-Sex Peer Groups," *Child Development* 74, no. 3 (2003): 921–932; Robert L. Munroe and A. Kimball Romney, "Gender and Age Differences in the Same-Sex Aggregation and Social Behaviors: A Four-Culture Study," *Journal of Cross-Cultural Psychology* 37, no. 1 (2006): 3–19.

111. Ballif-Spanvill et al., "Good Ole Boys."

112. Joyce F. Benenson and Kiran Alavi, "Sex Differences in Children's Investment in Same-Sex Peers," *Evolution and Human Behavior* 25, no. 4 (2004): 258–266.

125. Mark Bennett, Martyn Barrett, Rauf Karakozov, Giorgi Kipiani, Evanthia Lyons, Valentina Pavlenko, and Tatiana Riazanova, "Young Children's Evaluations of the Ingroup and of Outgroups: A Multi-national study," *Social Development* 13, no. 1 (2004): 124–141.

126. Mark Van Vugt, David De Cremer, and Dirk P. Janssen, "Gender Differences in Cooperation and Competition: The Male-Warrior Hypothesis," *Psychological Science* 18, no. 1 (2007): 19–23.

127. Ervin Staub, *The Roots of Evil: The Origins of Genocide and Other Group Violence* (New York: Cambridge University Press, 1989).

128. Goldstein, "Gender in the IR Textbook and Beyond."

129. Donelson R. Forsyth, *Group Dynamics*, 4th ed. (Belmont, CA: Thomson Wadsworth, 2006).

130. Gerben A. van Kleef, Christopher Oveis, Ilmo van der Löwe, Aleksandr Luo-Kogan, Jennifer Goetz, and Dacher Keltner, "Power, Distress, and Compassion: Turning a Blind Eye to the Suffering of Others," *Psychological Science* 19, no. 12 (2008): 1315–1322.

131. Nathanael J. Fast and Serena Chen, "When the Boss Feels Inadequate: Power, Incompetence, and Aggression," *Psychological Science* 20, no. 11 (2009): 1406–1413, doi: 10.1111/j.1467–9280.2009.02452.x.

132. Julia C. Babcock, Jennifer Waltz, Neil S. Jacobson, and John M. Gottman, "Power and Violence: The Relation Between Communication Patterns, Power Discrepancies, and Domestic Violence," *Journal of Consulting and Clinical Psychology* 61, no. 1 (1993): 40–50.

133. Ronald L. Akers, Marvin D. Krohn, Lonn Lanza-Kaduce, and Maria Radosevich, "Social Learning and Deviant Behavior: A Specific Test of a General Theory," *American Sociological Review* 44, no. 4 (1979): 636–655; Dana L. Haynie, "Delinquent Peers Revisited: Does Network Structure Matter?" *American Journal of Sociology* 106, no. 4 (2001): 1013–1057; Cesar J. Rebellon, "Do Adolescents Engage in Delinquency to Attract the Social Attention of Peers? An Extension of a Longitudinal Test of the Social Reinforcement Hypothesis," *Journal of Research in Crime and Delinquency* 43, no. 4 (2006): 387–411; Christine S. Sellers, John K. Cochran, and Katherine A. Branch, "Social Learning Theory and Partner Violence: A Research Note," *Deviant Behavior* 26, no. 4 (2005): 379–395.

134. Deborah M. Capaldi, Thomas J. Dishion, Mike Stoolmiller, and Karen Yoerger, "Aggression Toward Female Partners by At-Risk Young Men: The Contribution of Male Adolescent Friendships," *Developmental Psychology* 37, no. 1 (2001): 61–73; Stephen E. Humphrey and Arnold S. Kahn, "Fraternities, Athletic Teams, and Rape: Importance of Identification with a Risky Group,"

144. Gregory A. Raymond, "International Norms: Normative Orders and Peace," in J. A. Vasquez, ed., *What Do We Know About War*, 290 (New York: Rowman and Littlefield, 2000).

145. Gerald M. Erchak, "Family Violence," in Carol R. Ember and Melvin Ember, eds., *Research Frontiers in Anthropology* (Englewood Cliffs, NJ: Prentice-Hall, 1994); Gerald M. Erchak and Richard Rosenfeld, "Societal Isolations, Violent Norms, and Gender Relations: A Re-examination and Extension of Levinson's Model of Wife Beating," *Cross-Cultural Research* 28, no. 2 (1994): 111–133; David Levinson, *Family Violence in Cross-Cultural Perspective* (Newbury Park, CA: Sage, 1989); Cynthia Cockburn, "The Gendered Dynamics of Armed Conflict and Political Violence," in Caroline Moser and Fiona C. Clark, eds., *Victims, Perpetrators or Actors?: Gender, Armed Conflict, and Political Violence*, 13–29 (New York: Zed Books, 2001).

146. Jean Bethke Elshtain, *Women and War* (New York: Basic Books, 1987); Susan Brownmiller, *Against Our Will: Men, Women, and Rape* (New York: Simon and Schuster, 1975); Betty Reardon, *Sexism and the War System* (New York: Teachers College Press, 1985); Sara Ruddick, "Pacifying the Forces: Drafting Women in the Interests of Peace," *Signs* 8, no. 3 (1983): 470–489.

147. Mary Caprioli, "Primed for Violence: The Role of Gender Inequality in Predicting Internal Conflict," *International Studies Quarterly* 49, no. 2 (2005): 161–178.

148. Johan Galtung, *Peace: Research, Education, Action: Essays in Peace Research*, vol. 1 (Bucharest: CIPEXIM, 1990); Johan Galtung, "Cultural Violence," *Journal of Peace Research* 27, no. 3 (1990): 291–305.

149. Galtung, *Peace*, 80.

150. Ibid., 264–265.

151. Galtung, "Cultural Violence," 291.

152. Caprioli et al., "The WomanStats Database."

153. V. Spike Peterson, "Gendered National: Reproducing 'Us' Versus 'Them,'" in L.A. Lorentzen and J. Turpin, eds., *The Women and War Reader*, 42–43 (New York: New York University Press, 1998).

154. J. Ann Tickner, *Gender in International Relations: Feminist Perspectives on Achieving Global Security* (New York: Columbia University Press, 1992); Hanna Papanek, "To Each Less Than She Needs, From Each More Than She Can Do: Allocations, Entitlements, and Value," in Irene Tinker, ed., *Persistent Inequalities: Women and World Development*, 162–181 (New York and Oxford: Oxford University Press, 1994); Mark Tessler and Ina Warriner, "Gender, Feminism, and Attitudes Toward International Conflict," *World Politics* 49 (January 1997): 250–281; Caprioli, "Primed for Violence"; J. Ann Tickner, *Gendering World Politics* (New York: Columbia University Press, 2001).

7. Robert Kurzban, John Tooby, and Leda Cosmides, "Can Race Be 'Erased'? Coalitional Computation and Social Categorization," *Proceedings of the National Academy of Sciences* 98, no. 22 (2001): 15387–15392.

8. Quoted in Andrew Stephen, "Hating Hillary," *New Statesman*, May 22, 2008, www.newstatesman.com/north-america/2008/05/obama-clinton-vote-usa-media, accessed June 10, 2008.

9. Jacques Derrida, *Of Grammatology* (Baltimore: Johns Hopkins University Press, 1976); Jacques Derrida, *Writing and Difference* (London: Routledge, 1978).

10. We recognize that people in nearly every society, modern and historical, have found ways to modify their assigned gender. However, this involves a very small minority of people, with gender assignment being otherwise immutable for the overwhelming majority of society (Ramaswami Mahalingam, Jana Haritatos, and Benita Jackson, "Essentialism and the Cultural Psychology of Gender in Extreme Son Preference Communities in India," *American Journal of Orthopsychiatry* 77, no. 4 [October 2007]: 598–609).

11. Joseph Lopreato, *Human Nature and Biocultural Evolution* (Boston: Allen and Unwin, 1984); Richard Wrangham and Dale Peterson, *Demonic Males: Apes and the Origins of Human Violence* (New York: Houghton Mifflin, 1996).

12. Sylviane Agacinski, *The Parity of the Sexes* (New York: Columbia University Press, 2001), 14.

13. Eva M. Rathgeber, "WID, WAD, GAD: Trends in Research and Practice," *Journal of Developing Areas* 24, no. 4 (1990): 489–502; Martha Chen, "A Matter of Survival: Women's Right to Work in India and Bangladesh," in Martha Nussbaum and Jonathon Glover, eds., *Women and Culture and Development: A Study of Human Capabilities* (Oxford: Clarendon Press, 1992), 37–60; Jodi L. Jacobson, *Gender Bias: Roadblock to Sustainable Development* (Washington, DC: Worldwatch Institute, 1992); Amartya Sen, "Women's Survival as a Development Problem," *Bulletin of the American Academy of Arts and Sciences* 43 (1989): 14–29; Geeta Chowdery and Sheila Nair, *Power, Postcolonialism, and International Relations: Reading Race, Gender, and Class* (New York: Routledge, 2002).

14. World Economic Forum, "The Global Gender Gap Report," www.weforum.org/pdf/gendergap/report2007.pdf, accessed December 2007; World Bank, "Engendering Development: Through Gender Equality in Rights, Resources, and Voice," *World Bank Policy Research Report* (Washington, DC: Oxford University Press, 2001); John Hoddinott and Lawrence Haddad, "Does Female Income Share Influence Household Expenditure Patterns?" *Oxford Bulletin of Economics and Statistics* 57, no. 1 (2001): 77–97.

15. Duncan Thomas, "Intrahousehold Resource Allocation: An Inferential Approach," *Journal of Human Resources* 25 (1990): 635–664; Duncan Thomas, Dante Contreras, and Elizabeth Frankenberg, *Child Health and the Distribu-

2002); J. Ann Tickner, *Gender in International Relations: Feminist Perspectives on Achieving Global Security* (New York: Columbia University Press, 1992); J. Ann Tickner, *Gendering World Politics* (New York: Columbia University Press, 2001); J. Ann Tickner, "Hans Morgenthau's Principles of Political Realism: A Feminist Reformulation," *Millennium: Journal of International Studies* 17, no. 3 (1998): 429–440; Rebecca Grant and Kathleen Newland, *Gender and International Relations* (Bloomington: Indiana University Press, 1991); Jan Jindy Pettman, *Worlding Women: A Feminist International Politics* (New York: Routledge, 1996); Marysia Zalewski and Jane Papart, eds., *The "Man" Question in International Relations* (Boulder, CO: Lynne Rienner Publishers, 1998); see also Francis Fukuyama, "Women and the Evolution of World Politics," *Foreign Affairs* 77, no. 5 (September/October 1998): 24–40. A new generation continues this important tradition; see, for example, Laura Sjoberg, ed., *Gender and International Relations: Feminist Perspectives* (New York: Routledge, 2009); Laura Shepherd, ed., *Gender Matters in Global Politics: A Feminist Introduction to International Relations* (New York: Routledge, 2010); Natalie Florea Hudson, *Gender, Human Security, and the United Nations: Security Language as a Political Framework for Women* (New York: Routledge, 2009), to cite but a few such works.

21. Swanee Hunt and Cristina Posa, "Women Waging Peace," *Foreign Policy* (May/June 2001): 38–47; Natalie Florea Hudson, "Securitizing Women and Gender Equality: Who and What Is It Good For?" (paper presented at the International Studies Association, Chicago, March 2007); see also www.peacewomen.org.

22. J. Ann Tickner, "What Is Your Research Program? Some Feminist Answers to IR's Methodological Questions," *International Studies Quarterly* 49, no. 1 (2005): 1–21; V. Spike Peterson, "(On) The Cutting Edge: Feminist Research in International Relations" (presentation at the University of Arizona Association for Women Faculty Meeting, Tucson, February 1991); Sylvester, "'Progress' as Feminist International Relations"; Jill Steans, "Engaging from the Margins: Feminist Encounters with the 'Mainstream' of International Relations," *British Journal of Politics and International Relations* 5, no. 3 (2003): 428–454.

23. See, for example, Lene Hansen, *Security as Practice: Discourse Analysis and the Bosnian War* (New York: Routledge, 2006); Sandra Whitworth, *Men, Militarism, and UN Peacekeeping* (Boulder, CO: Lynne Rienner Publishers, 2004); Dubravka Zarkov, *The Body of War: Media, Ethnicity, and Gender in the Break-up of Yugoslavia* (Durham, NC: Duke University Press, 2007); Dyan Mazurana, Angela Raven-Roberts, and Jane Parpart, eds., *Gender, Conflict, and Peacekeeping* (New York: Rowman and Littlefield, 2005).

24. Sylvester, *Feminist International Relations*.

36. Natalie B. Florea, Mark A. Boyer, Scott W. Brown, Michael J. Butler, Magnolia Hernandez, Kimberly Weir, Lin Meng, Paula R. Johnson, Clarisse Lima, and Hayley J. Mayall, "Negotiating from Mars to Venus: Gender in Simulated International Negotiations," *Simulation and Gaming* 34, no. 2 (2003): 226–248.

37. Huntington, *The Clash of Civilizations and the Remaking of World Order*.

38. Ronald Ingelhart and Pippa Norris, "The True Clash of Civilizations," *Foreign Policy* 135 (March/April 2003): 63–70; Ronald Ingelhart and Pippa Norris, *Rising Tide: Gender Equality and Cultural Change Around the World* (New York: Cambridge University Press, 2003).

39. Martha Nussbaum, *Women and Human Development: The Capabilities Approach* (Cambridge: Cambridge University Press, 2000); Martha Nussbaum, "Human Capabilities, Female Human Beings," in Martha Nussbaum and Jonathon Glover, eds., *Women, Culture, and Development*, 61–104 (New York: Oxford University Press, 1995).

40. David L. Cingranelli and David L. Richards, "The Cingranelli-Richards (CIRI) Human Rights Dataset," version 2006.10.02, www.humanrightsdata.org.

41. UNECA, "The African Gender and Development Index," available at www.uneca.org/eca_programmes/acgd/publications/agdi_book_final.pdf, 2005, accessed July 24, 2007.

42. Mary Caprioli, Valerie M. Hudson, Rose McDermott, Bonnie Ballif-Spanvill, Chad F. Emmett, and S. Matthew Stearmer, "The WomanStats Project Database: Advancing an Empirical Research Agenda," *Journal of Peace Research* 46, no. 6 (November 2009): 1–13.

43. The data are freely accessible to anyone with an Internet connection (www.womanstats.org), thus facilitating worldwide scholarship on these issues. Contribution of data via remote upload is also possible for approved credentialed sources.

44. Good primers on polytomous logistic regression, sometimes called ordinal regression, are available here: Marija Norusis, "Ordinal Regression," in her book *SPSS Advanced Statistical Procedures Companion* (New York: Prentice Hall, 2010), 69–89, www.norusis.com/pdf/ASPC_v13.pdf; and also Richard Williams, "Statistics II: Ordered Logit Models—Overview" (Department of Sociology, University of Notre Dame, n.d.), www.nd.edu/~rwilliam/stats2/l91.pdf.

45. To test the civilizational explanation for state peacefulness, a particular identity associated with greater levels of conflict or a lack of state peacefulness must first be identified. In the early years of the twenty-first century, Islamic civilization—rightly or wrongly—has been singled out for this dubious distinction (see, for example, Lee Harris, *Civilization and Its Enemies: The Next Stage of History* (New York: Free Press, 2004); Norman Podhoretz, *World War IV: The*

5. WINGS OF NATIONAL AND INTERNATIONAL RELATIONS, PART ONE

1. V. Spike Peterson, "Security and Sovereign States: What Is at Stake in Taking Feminism Seriously?" in V. Spike Peterson, ed., *Gendered States: Feminist (Re)Visions of International Relations Theory* (Boulder, CO: Lynne Rienner Publishers, 1992), 31–64.

2. We thank *Foreign Policy* magazine for permission to use material from our article Valerie M. Hudson and Patricia Leidl, "Betrayed," *Foreign Policy*, May 10, 2010, www.foreignpolicy.com/articles/2010/05/07/the_us_is_abandoning _afghanistan_s_women?page=0,0, accessed May 22, 2010.

3. Hudson and Leidl, "Betrayed."

4. Wheatley Institution, Brigham Young University, Provo, Utah, March 26, 2010.

5. "Subjugation of Women Is Threat to US Security: Clinton," *Agence France-Presse*, March 12, 2010, www.google.com/hostednews/afp/article/ALeqM5ib71t2 EuWmwDahxNKDaHxcEbfcYA, accessed May 18, 2010.

6. V. Spike Peterson, ed., *Gendered States: Feminist (Re)Visions of International Relations Theory* (Boulder, CO: Lynne Rienner Publishers, 1992); V. Spike Peterson, "Gendered National: Reproducing 'Us' Versus 'Them,'" in Lois A. Lorentzen and Jennifer Turpin, eds., *The Women and War Reader* (New York: New York University Press, 1998), 41–49

7. Arthur N. Gilbert and James F. Cole, "Revolutionary Theory and Gender Theory: The Iranian Case" (paper prepared for the International Studies Association annual conference, Chicago, February 21–25, 1995), 12.

8. CNN, "New Protest Statement Builds in Iran—Men in Head Scarves," December 14, 2009, http://edition.cnn.com/2009/WORLD/meast/12/14/iran.head scarf.protest/, accessed May 18, 2010.

9. UN Treaties, http://treaties.un.org/Pages/ViewDetails.aspx?src=IND&mtdsg_ no=IV-8&chapter=4&lang=en, accessed May 18, 2010.

10. UN Treaties, http://treaties.un.org/Pages/ViewDetails.aspx?src=TREATY& mtdsg_no=IV-8&chapter=4&lang=en, accessed May 18, 2010.

11. "Grassroots Politics and Women's Activism Forum in D.C.," Muslimahmediawatch, November 17, 2009, http://muslimahmediawatch.org/2009/11/grass roots-politics-and-womens-activism-forum-in-d-c/, accessed May 18, 2010.

12. "Understanding Islamic Feminism: An Interview with Ziba Mir-Hosseini, February 7, 2010, http://madrasareforms.blogspot.com/2010/02/understanding-islamic-feminism.html, accessed May 18, 2010.

13. "Middle East: Regional Coalition 'Equality Without Reservation,'" Women Living Under Muslim Laws, n.d., www.wluml.org/node/4563, accessed May 18, 2010.

27. Kristine Pearson of Lifeline Energy (http://lifelineenergy.org) (remarks presented at the Radcliffe Institute conference "Driving Change, Shaping Lives: Gender in the Developing World," Cambridge, MA, March 3–4, 2011).

28. Marilyn Waring, *Counting for Nothing: What Men Value and What Women Are Worth*, (2nd ed., Toronto: University of Toronto Press, 2004).

29. Office of the High Commissioner for Human Rights, "Project on a Mechanism to Address Laws That Discriminate Against Women.," March 6, 2008, www .ohchr.org/Documents/Publications/laws_that_discriminate_against_women .pdf, accessed May 18, 2010.

30. BBC, "New Poster to Attack Prostitution," May 5, 2008, http://news.bbc .co.uk/2/hi/uk_news/7384006.stm, accessed May 18, 2010.

31. Julie Bindel, "Iceland: The World's Most Feminist Country," *Guardian*, March 25, 2010, www.guardian.co.uk/lifeandstyle/2010/mar/25/iceland-most-feminist-country, accessed May 18, 2010.

32. Jeanne Sarson and Linda MacDonald, "Defining Torture by Non-State Actors in the Canadian Private Sphere," *First Light*, Winter 2009, 29–33, www.ccvt .org/pdfs/firstlighwinter2009.pdf, accessed May 18, 2010.

33. Julia Preston, "New Policy Permits Asylum for Battered Women," *New York Times*, July 15, 2009, www.nytimes.com/2009/07/16/us/16asylum.html?_r=1&scp =1&sq=asylum%20domestic%20violence&st=cse, accessed May 18, 2010.

34. Bruce Crumley, "French Bid to Ban Marital Abuse That's Psychological," *Time*, January 9, 2010, www.time.com/time/world/article/0,8599,1952552,00 .html, accessed May 18, 2010.

35. WUNRN, "Sierra Leone Judgment on Forced Marriage," March 23, 2009, www .wunrn.com/news/2009/03_09/03_23_09/032309_sierra.html, accessed May 18, 2010.

36. Una Hombrecher, "Overcoming Domestic Violence" (Stuttgart: Social Service Agency of the Protestant Church in Germany, 2007), 68, www2.wcc-coe.org/dov .nsf/41c6b7355083931ec1256c14002d2a77/6714af73bd48efe9c12574aa003d0616/ $FILE/BfdW-BUCHHuslGewENGL_final2.pdf, accessed May 18, 2010.

37. Robert Jensen (remarks at the Radcliffe Institute conference "Driving Change, Shaping Lives: Gender in the Developing World," Cambridge, MA, March 3–4, 2011). In another experiment, in which Jensen provided information, recruitment, and follow-up on job opportunities in the big cities for girls who were located in rural Indian communities, he found a significant increase in vaccination rates, school attendance, and even the weight of girls in the villages over three years. Again, envisioning a different life for girls is one of the first steps to greater family investment in girls.

would simply determine that they absolutely must be literate, and then have their children teach them basic literacy at home in a very short time.

47. Encyclopedia.com, "Court Bans Fatwas," February 2, 2001, www.encyclopedia .com/doc/1G1–71202881.html, accessed May 18, 2010.

48. Chris Kiwawulo, "Bride Price Petition, Uganda MIFUMI Court Case," *Mifumi*, April 7, 2010, http://mifumi.org/blog/?tag=bride-price-petition-uganda-mifumi-court-case, accessed May 18, 2010.

49. Paola Bergalla and Augustina Ramon Michel, "Argentina: Two Judicial Decisions Regarding Abortion in the Case of Rape" (Universidad de San Andres, April 19, 2010), www.wunrn.com/news/2010/04_10/04_19_10/041910_argentina .htm, accessed May 18, 2010.

50. Asia-Pacific Forum on Women, Law, and Development, "Negotiating Culture: Intersections of Culture and Violence Against Women in the Asia-Pacific," 2006, http://pacific.ohchr.org/docs/Culture_and_VAW-Final_Report_Oct_30_ (2).doc, accessed May 18, 2010.

51. Sara Israelson-Hartley and Wendy Leonard, "Talking About Religion May Solve the World's Big Problems," *Deseret News*, November 22, 2009, www .deseretnews.com/article/705346068/Talking-about-religion-may-solve-worlds-big-problems.html?pg=2, accessed May 18, 2010.

52. Ann Jones, "The Terrifying Normalcy of Assaulting Women," *Alternet*, May 14, 2008, www.alternet.org/reproductivejustice/85282?page=entire, accessed May 18, 2010.

53. Elaine Ganley, "France: Polygamy Banned, but Complex Issues," Human Rights Without Frontiers, May 3, 2010, www.wunrn.com/news/2010/05_10/05_ 03_10/050310_france.htm, accessed May 18, 2010.

54. Women Living Under Muslim Laws, "UK: Muslim Institute Launches New Model Muslim Marriage Contract," August 11, 2008, www.wluml.org/node/ 4749, accessed May 18, 2010.

55. Harry Eckstein, A *Theory of Stable Democracy* (Princeton, NJ: Center of International Studies, Woodrow Wilson School of Public and International Affairs, Princeton University, 1961), iii, http://hdl.handle.net/2027/mdp .39015008254560.

56. Frances Harrison, "Egypt Bans 92-Year Old's Marriage," *BBC News*, June 13, 2008, http://news.bbc.co.uk/2/hi/7452456.stm, accessed May 18, 2010.

57. PhilGAD Portal, "PGMA Signs Magna Carta of Women," Philippine Commission on Women, August 14, 2009, www.ncrfw.gov.ph/index.php/ncrfw-press-releases/349-news-ncrfw-pgma-signs-mcw, accessed May 18, 2010.

58. Guatemalan Human Rights Commission, "Guatemala's Femicide Law: Progress Against Impunity?" 2009, www.ghrc-usa.org/Publications/Femicide_Law_ ProgressAgainstImpunity.pdf, accessed May 18, 2010.

73. Steven Erlanger, "For Women Who Lead, a Forum of Their Own," *New York Times*, October 19, 2008, www.nytimes.com/2008/10/20/world/europe/20france .html, accessed May 18, 2010.

74. Donald Steinberg, "Combating Sexual Violence in Conflict: Using Facts from the Ground" (address to the United Nations, December 17, 2008), www.wunrn .com/news/2009/01_09/01_12_09/011209_combating.htm, accessed May 18, 2010.

75. Measure Evaluation, "Violence Against Women and Girls: A Compendium of Monitoring and Evaluation Indicators," n.d., www.cpc.unc.edu/measure/tools/ gender/violence-against-women-and-girls-compendium-of-indicators; see also Report of the Secretary-General, United Nations, "Women and Peace and Security," April 6, 2010, www.un.org/ga/search/view_doc.asp?symbol=S/2010/173, accessed May 18, 2010.

76. Lizette Alvarez, "Sweden Faces Facts on Violence Against Women," *New York Times*, March 30, 2005, www.nytimes.com/2005/03/29/world/europe/29iht-letter-4909045.html?pagewanted=1&emc=eta1, accessed May 18, 2010.

77. "Peace and Security for All" (Feminist Institute of the Heinrich Boll Foundation, May 2006), www.boell.de/publications/feminism-gender-democracy-8878.html, accessed June 1, 2010.

78. Nobel Women's Initiative Conference, "Women Redefining Democracy" (Antigua, Guatemala, May 10–12, 2009), www.nobelwomensinitiative.org/search/ results/post/redefining-democracy-declaration, accessed May 18, 2010.

6. WINGS OF NATIONAL AND INTERNATIONAL RELATIONS, PART TWO

1. Barry Schwartz, "In 'Sticky' Ideas, More Is Less," *Washington Post*, January 17, 2007, www.washingtonpost.com/wp-dyn/content/article/2007/01/16/ AR2007011601625.html, accessed May 27, 2010.

2. Some of our favorite such groups include GirlEffect, Women for Women International, and Equality Now, but there are many fine groups worldwide. Peacewomen.org provides a very detailed list of both indigenous and transnational groups working for a better situation for women and girls. Another excellent source of information on local groups and their efforts is the Women News Network video collection, at http://womennewsnetwork.vodpod.com/. Our own project website, Womanstats.org , is a critical piece of infrastructure for chronicling the situation of women; our home page at www.womanstats.org provides information on how to support our research, through donating either time or funds.

3. Donna Abu-Nasr, "Saudi Girls Should Be Allowed to Play Sports, Says Prince," *Huffington Post*, June 23, 2009, www.huffingtonpost.com/2009/06/23/saudi-girls-should-be-all_n_219692.html, accessed May 27, 2010.

16. Ed Vulliamy, "Breaking the Silence," *Guardian*, October 5, 2005, www.guard ian.co.uk/media/2005/oct/05/broadcasting.saudiarabia, accessed May 27, 2010.

17. "My Mother Held Me Down," *BBC News*, July 10, 2007, http://news.bbc.co .uk/2/hi/health/6287926.stm, accessed May 27, 2010.

18. Waris Dirie Foundation, "About Waris Dirie," 2010, www.waris-dirie-foundation .com/en/about-waris-dirie/, accessed May 27, 2010.

19. HBDGWerbeagentur. "Waris Dirie: Stop FGM Now" (video file), February 5, 2010, Retrieved from http://adsoftheworld.com/media/tv/waris_dirie_ stop_fgm_now, accessed May 27, 2010.

20. Middle East Media Research Institute (MEMRI), "Saudi Cleric, Women's Rights Activist in TV Debate on Types of Marriage in Arab World (special dispatch no. 2144), December 8, 2008, www.memri.org/report/en/0/0/0/0/0/0/2979 .htm, accessed May 27, 2010.

21. Katherine Zoepf, "Saudi Women Find an Unlikely Role Model: Oprah," *New York Times*, September 19, 2008, www.nytimes.com/2008/09/19/world/ middleeast/19oprah.html?scp=1&sq=zoepf%20saudi%20oprah&st=cse.

22. Jamel Arfaoui, "New Tunisian Film Calls Attention to Inheritance Law," *Magharebia*, August 10, 2008, www.magharebia.com/cocoon/awi/xhtml1/en_ GB/features/awi/features/2008/10/08/feature-01, accessed May 27, 2010.

23. Nazila Fathi. "Starting at Home: Iran's Women Fight for Rights," *New York Times*, February 12, 2009, www.nytimes.com/2009/02/13/world/middleeast/ 13iran.html?scp=1&sq=nazila%20fathi%202009%20starting%20at%20home&st =cse, accessed May 27, 2010.

24. journeymanpictures, "Iran's Fearless Film Maker" (video file), February 4, 2008, www.youtube.com/watch?v=QFIjKBsuZTQ&feature=fvw, accessed May 27, 2010.

25. Tahmineh Milani, Internet Movie Database, www.imdb.com/name/nm 0586841/, accessed May 27, 2010.

26. "New Films to Debut at Iranian Theaters in Noruz," *Tehran Times*, March 9, 2010, www.tehrantimes.com/index.asp?newspaper_no=10826&B1=View+the+ newspapr, accessed May 27, 2010.

27. "The Seventh Biennial Conference on Iranian studies: Toronto, Canada, July 31– August 3, 2008," *Payvand*, http://payvand.com/news/08/jun/1066.html, accessed May 27, 2010.

28. Fathi, "Starting at Home."

29. "Saudi Women Make Video Protest," *BBC News*, March 11, 2008, http://news .bbc.co.uk/2/hi/middle_east/7159077.stm, accessed May 27, 2010.

30. "Saudi Women Challenge Driving Ban," *BBC News*, September 18, 2007, http:// news.bbc.co.uk/2/hi/middle_east/7000499.stm, accessed May 27, 2010.

43. Mark Lacey, "Genital Cutting Shows Signs of Losing Favor in Africa," *New York Times*, June 8, 2004, www.nytimes.com/2004/06/08/international/africa/08 cutt.html?scp=2&sq=lacey%20genital%20cutting%20favor%20africa&st=cse, accessed May 27, 2010.

44. "Experts: Black Church Can Better Address Domestic Violence," Weblog entry, *ReligionNewsBlog*, September 10, 2007, www.religionnewsblog.com/19324/domestic-violence-3, accessed May 27, 2010.

45. Yigal Schliefer, "In Turkey, Muslim Women Gain Expanded Religious Authority," *Christian Science Monitor*, April 27, 2005, www.csmonitor.com/2005/0427/p04s01-woeu.html, accessed May 27, 2010.

46. Kwame Anthony Appiah, "The Art of Social Change," *New York Times*, October 22, 2010, www.nytimes.com/2010/10/24/magazine/24FOB-Footbinding-t.html, accessed 1 March 2011.

47. Quoted in Doron Shultziner and Mary Ann Tetreault, "Paradoxes of Democratic Progress in Kuwait: The Case of the Kuwaiti Women's Rights Movement," *Muslim World Journal of Human Rights* 7, no. 2 (2011): 17.

48. Stephanie Hancock, "Creating a Woman's World in Arabia," *BBC News*, March 4, 2009, http://news.bbc.co.uk/2/hi/middle_east/7922279.stm, accessed May 27, 2010.

49. Michael Slackman, "Sidewalks, and an Identity, Sprout in Jordan's Capital, *New York Times*, February 23, 2010, www.nytimes.com/2010/02/24/world/middleeast/24amman.html?scp=1&sq=slackman%20sidewalks%20jordan&st=cse, accessed May 27, 2010.

50. Huma Yusuf, "People Making a Difference: Sheema Kermani," *Christian Science Monitor*, June 8, 2009, www.csmonitor.com/The-Culture/Home/2009/0608/p47s01-lihc.html, accessed May 27, 2010.

51. Tom Engelhardt, "Tomgram: Ann Jones, Changing the World One Shot at a Time," *TomDispatch.com*, May 13, 2008, www.tomdispatch.com/post/174931, accessed May 27, 2010.

52. Abdullah Nasser al-Fouzan, "Moudhi Riding on a Donkey," *Saudi Gazette*, May 29, 2010, www.saudigazette.com.sa/index.cfm?method=home.regcon&contentID=2010040168079, accessed May 29, 2010. Some have suggested this story is apocryphal, while others insist it is true. The fact that such a story is still circulating shows its deep resonance within the culture.

53. Isabel Kershner, "On One Field, Two Goals: Equality and Statehood," *New York Times*, October 28, 2009, www.nytimes.com/2009/10/29/world/middleeast/29westbank.html?scp=1&sq=kershner%20one%20field%20two%20goals&st=cse, accessed May 27, 2010.

54. Women for Women International, "Ending Violence Against Women in Eastern Congo: Preparing Men to Advocate for Women's Rights," 2007, www

65. Emily Wax, "In India, New Seat of Power for Women," *Washington Post*, October 12, 2009, www.washingtonpost.com/wp-dyn/content/article/2009/10/11/AR2009101101934.html, accessed May 27, 2010.

66. Fathi, "Starting at Home."

67. Robert F. Worth, "Arab TV Tests Societies' Limits with Depictions of Sex and Equality," *New York Times*, September 2008, 26, www.nytimes.com/2008/09/27/world/middleeast/27beirut.html?scp=1&sq=arab%20tv%20tests%20depictions%20sex%20equality&st=cse, accessed May 27, 2010.

68. Karin Laub and Dalia Nammari, "Soap Opera Shakes Customs of Arab Married Life," *USA Today*, July 27, 2008, www.usatoday.com/life/television/2008–07–27–733717293_x.htm , accessed May 27, 2010.

69. Hunt Alternatives Fund, "Asha Hagi Elmi: Expert Spotlight," April 2007, www.huntalternatives.org/download/498_4_26_07_somali_woman_leader_peace_cal.pdf, accessed May 27, 2010.

70. Susan McKay, "How Do You Mend Broken Hearts? Gender, War, and Impacts on Girls in Fighting Forces," in G. Reyes and G. A. Jacobs, eds., *Handbook of International Disaster Psychology*, 4:45–60 (Westport, CT: Praeger, 2006).

71. Iris Bohnet, "Gender Equality: A Nudge in the Right Direction," *Financial Times*, October 13, 2010, FT.com.

72. Bonnie Ballif-Spanvill, "The Most Critical Education for the 21st Century, Particularly for Girls and Women, Is Teaching People to Get Along with Each Other" (paper presented at the UN Commission on the Status of Women, New York, March 2010).

73. Interview with S. Matthew Stearmer, May 27, 2010.

74. Blaine Harden, "Learn to Be Nice to Your Wife, or Pay the Price," *Washington Post*, November 26, 2007, www.washingtonpost.com/wp-dyn/content/article/2007/11/25/AR2007112501720.html, accessed May 27, 2010.

75. Thomas L. Friedman, "Postcard from Yemen," *New York Times*, February 8, 2010, http://topics.nytimes.com/top/news/international/countriesandterritories/yemen/index.html?scp=1&sq=postcard%20from%20yemen&st=cse, accessed May 27, 2010.

76. Greg Mortenson and David Oliver Relin, *Three Cups of Tea: One Man's Mission to Promote Peace . . . One School at a Time* (New York: Penguin, 2006), 153.

77. Colleen Johnson, "The Social Problems That Deter Xhosa Women from Marriage and How Education and Westernization Allow Them to Refuse Marriage" (honors thesis, Brigham Young University, Provo, Utah, 2006), 9–10.

78. Michael Hall, "The Mechanics of Relations Submission," WomanStats Blog, September 17, 2009, womanstats.org/blog2nd09.htm#submission, accessed May 27, 2010, abridged with the permission of the author.

CONTRIBUTORS

VALERIE M. HUDSON is Professor and George H. W. Bush Chair in The Bush School of Government and Public Service at Texas A&M University, having previously taught at Brigham Young, Northwestern, and Rutgers universities. Her research foci include foreign policy analysis, security studies, gender and international relations, and methodology. Hudson's articles have appeared in such journals as *International Security*, *Journal of Peace Research*, *Political Psychology*, and *Foreign Policy Analysis*. She is the author or editor of several books, including (with Andrea Den Boer) *Bare Branches: The Security Implications of Asia's Surplus Male Population* (MIT Press, 2004), which won the American Association of Publishers Award for the Best Book in Political Science, and the Otis Dudley Duncan Award for Best Book in Social Demography, resulting in feature stories in the *New York Times*, the *Economist*, *60 Minutes*, and other news publications. Hudson was named to *Foreign Policy* magazine's list of Top 100 Global Thinkers for 2009.

BONNIE BALLIF-SPANVILL is an emeritus professor of psychology and was the last director of the Women's Research Institute at Brigham Young University. After twenty-five years as a professor and department chair in the graduate school of Fordham University at Lincoln Center in New York City, she returned to her alma mater in 1994. Her research publications and papers in human motivation and emotion earned her the Fellow status in both the American Psychological Association, in 1984, and the Association for Psychological Science, in 1987. Currently, she is studying the ramifications of violence and development of peace in women and men across ages and in different circumstances and cultures worldwide. Her recent publications address intergenerational domestic violence, the impact of witnessing violence, and the design of techniques to increase peacefulness. She has also published a global anthology of poetry by women, revealing their experiences with violence and their resilient visions of peace.

MARY CAPRIOLI is an associate professor and Head of political science and Director of International Studies at the University of Minnesota Duluth. She has researched the role of gendered structural inequality on political conflict and violence. Caprioli pioneered a new line of scholarly inquiry between the security of women and the national and international behavior of states and confirmed the link using quantitative methodology. Her expertise has been sought by scholars worldwide. She is an associate editor for *Foreign Policy Analysis*, is a member of the WomanStats board of directors, and is an advisory board member of the Minorities at Risk Project. She received her PhD from the University of Connecticut.

INDEX

and Sex Ratio Scale, 57; Trafficking in Females Scale, 58
sovereignty, 38–39
Spain, CEDAW, 124
sports, 158, 166, 168–169, 177
Sri Lanka: activism, 162; terrorism, 115
States of Concern to the International Community (SOCIC) scale, 107, 109–113
statistics on women, 104–106, 153, 206
Staub, Ervin, 89
Steinberg, Donald, 153
stereotypes, gender, 88, 98
sterilization, forced, 129–130
structural violence, 93–94
submission, relational, 196–197
Sudan, starvation, 27
suffrage, women's, 40, 139, 162, 168, 169, 174
suicide, 4, 28, 96–97, 117, 166; honor suicides, 10; rape victims, 160, 183; terrorism, 149
Sulabh International, 187
Sullivan, Kevin, 24
survivors of abuse, 10, 168, 183, 186
Susan B. Anthony and Frederick Douglass Prenatal Nondiscrimination Act (House Bill 1822), 260n38
Suzuki, David, 44
Swaziland, prostitutes, 25–26
Sweden: CEDAW, 124; domestic violence, 22, 153; Maternal Mortality Scale, 61; prostitution, terms used to describe, 136; Trafficking in Females Scale, 58
Switzerland: Discrepancy in Education Scale, 61, 62; right to vote, 40, 168; Son Preference and Sex Ratio Scale, 57
Syria, 140; Discrepancy in Education Scale, 62; honor killings, 36; Intermingling in Public in the Islamic World Scale, 64; men, activism by, 178; punishment for honor killings, 138
Syrian Women Observatory, 178

Taeuber, Irene, 51
Tahmasebi, Susan, 167
Tahrir Square, Egypt, 203

Taiwan: sex ratios, 28; Son Preference and Sex Ratio Scale, 57
Tajikistan, Required Codes of Dress for Women in the Islamic World, 67
Takrori, Rukayya, 177
Taliban, 21, 120–121, 150, 152, 207
tax regulations, 119–120
Taylor, Debbie, 150
TBAs (traditional birth attendants), 141, 260n46
teaching gender equality, 190–193
technology, 163–168
Tehrik-e-Niswan (Women's Movement), 175
television, 163–165, 187–188
terrorism, 115, 116, 118, 149
testimony of women in court, weight of, 35–36
testosterone levels, 45, 78
Tetreault, Mary Ann, 139, 174
Texas, United States: criminal punishment for "crimes of passion," 36; policymaking, 43
Thaqui, Behan, 10
Thatcher, Margaret, 42
Thayer, Bradley, 69, 76, 77, 85
theater, 175
theoretical concerns with research methods, 108–109
thinking patterns for avoiding gender conflicts, 180, 184–190
Three Cups of Tea (Mortenson), 193
Together for Women's Development, 182
toilets, 186–187
Tomaselli, Keyan, 86
top-down approaches to gender equality, 16, 119–156
torture, domestic violence as, 136
traditional birth attendants (TBAs), 141, 260n46
traditional societies, 29–32, 38–39, 129, 150
trafficking: regional patterns, 58; sex trafficking, 13; Trafficking in Females Scale, 57–58; Trafficking in Persons Report (State Department), 58, 134; Trafficking in Victims Protection Act of 2000, 58